Organ Donation and Transplantation

Edited by Vassil Mihaylov

Published in London, United Kingdom

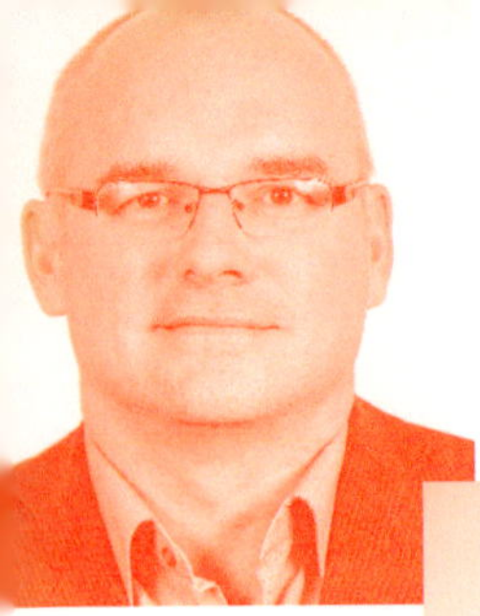
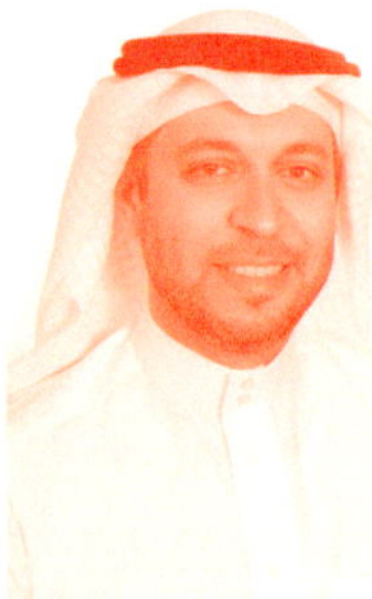
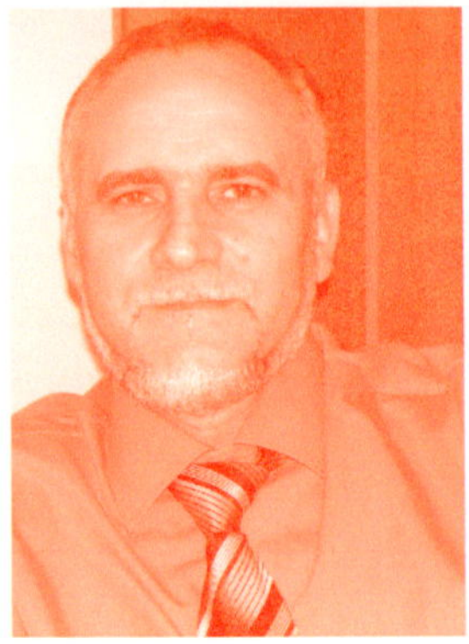
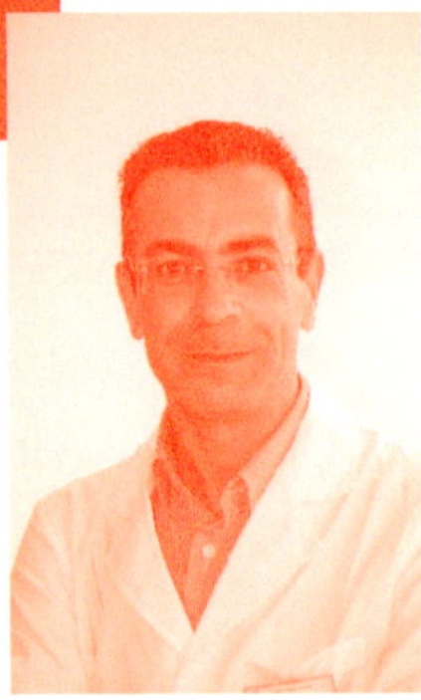
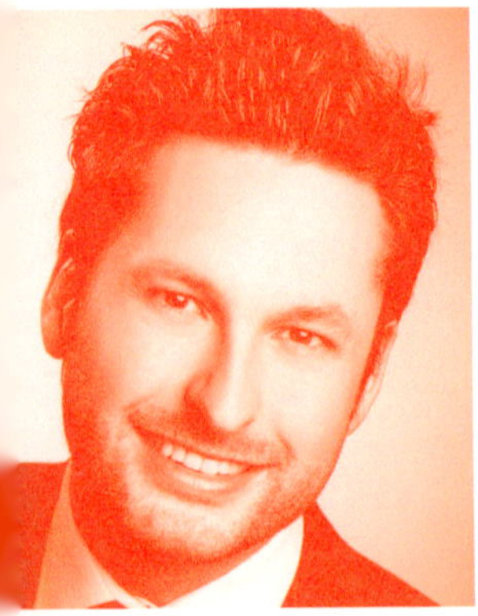
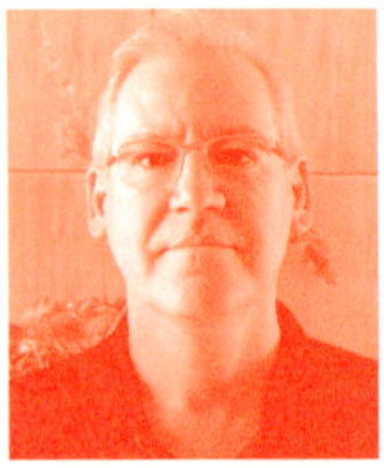
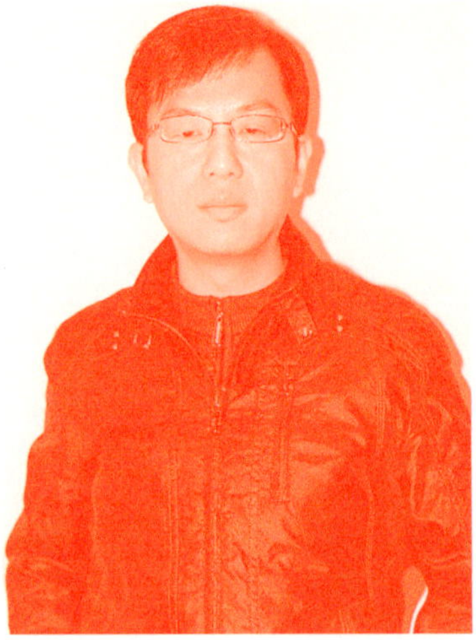

IntechOpen

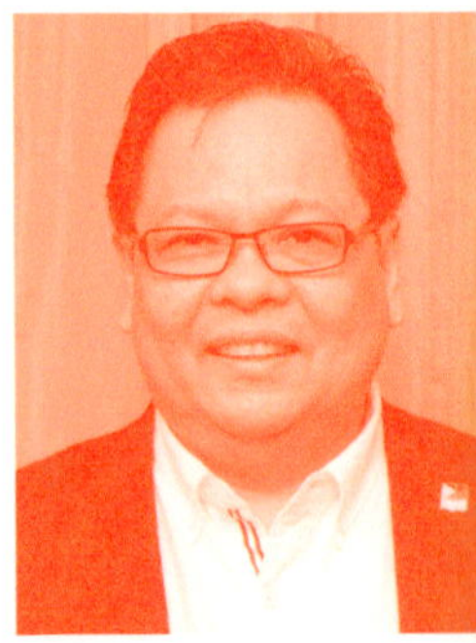
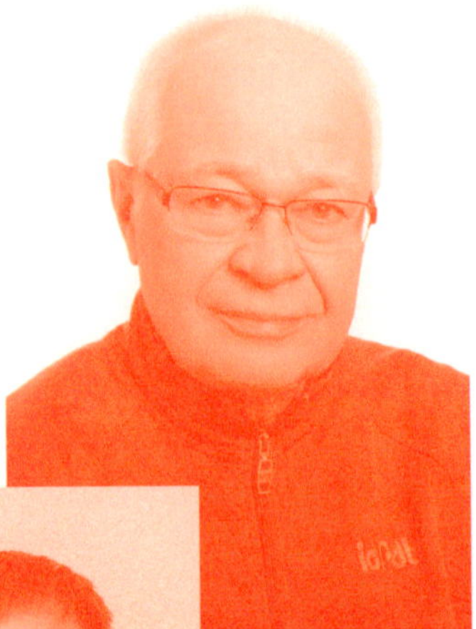
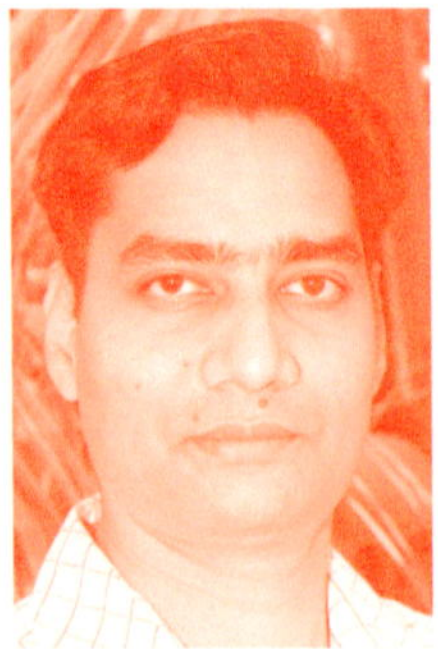
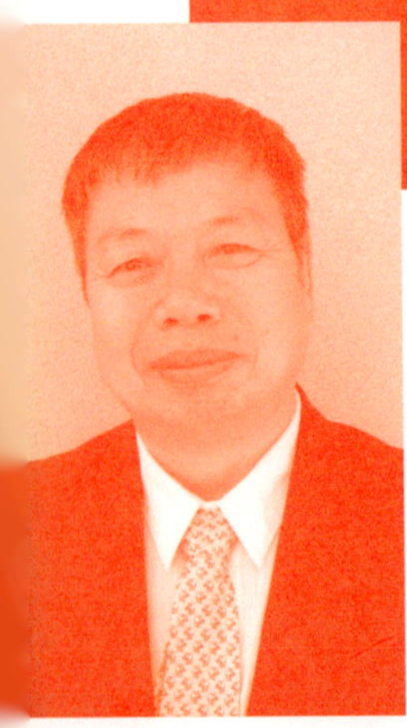
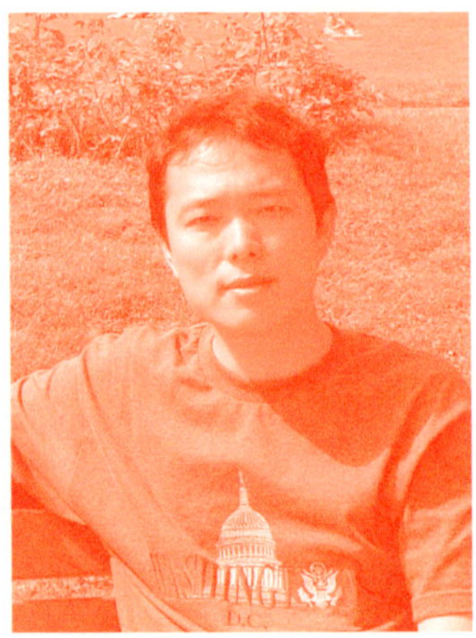
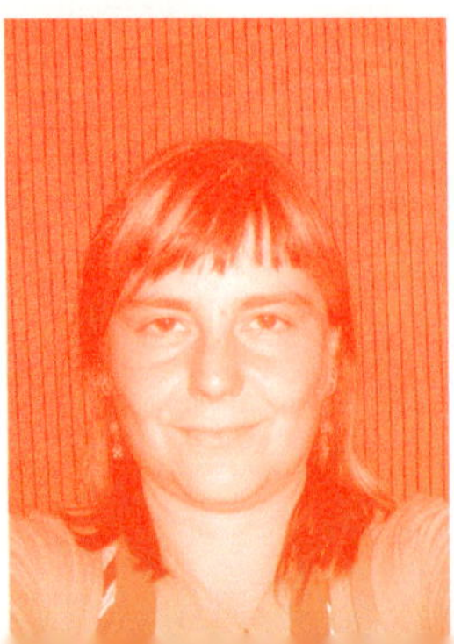

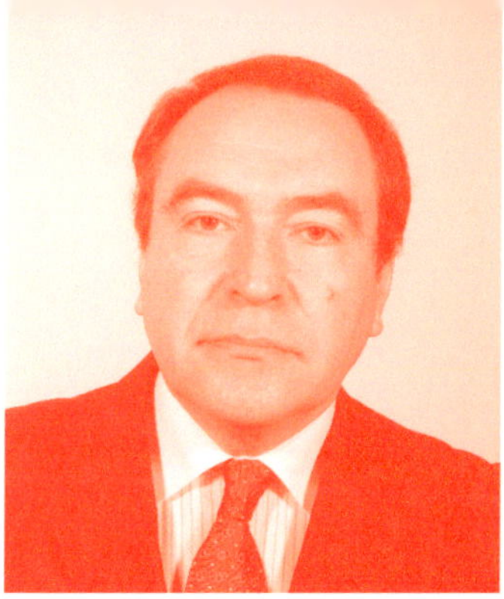

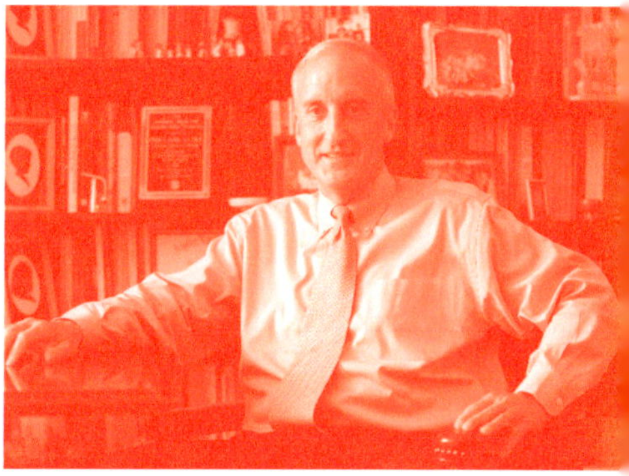

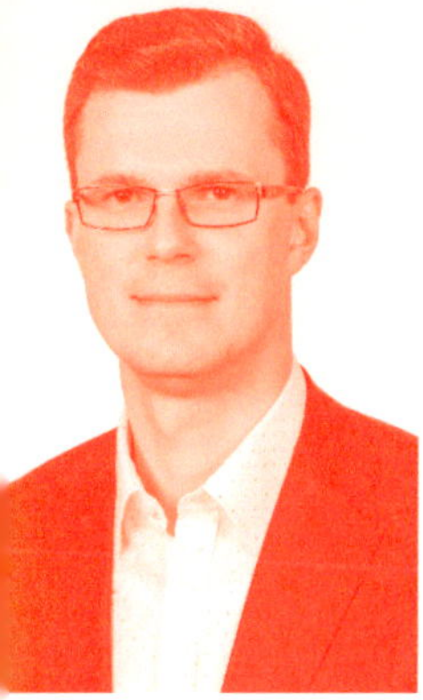

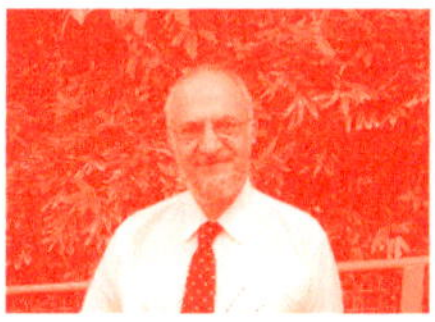

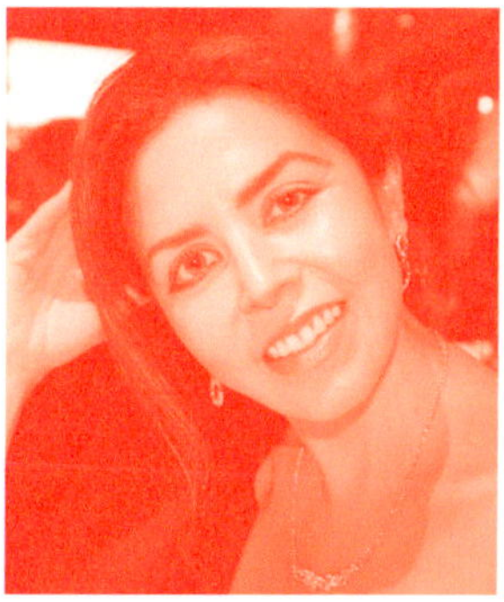

Supporting open minds since 2005

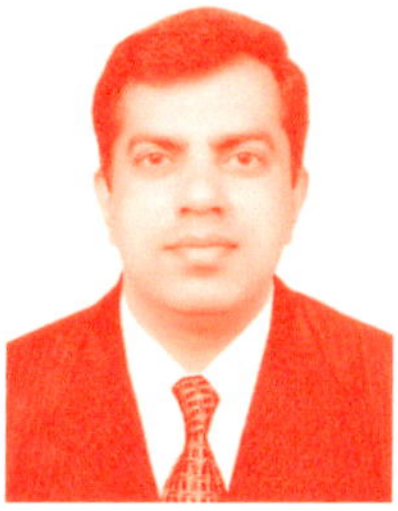

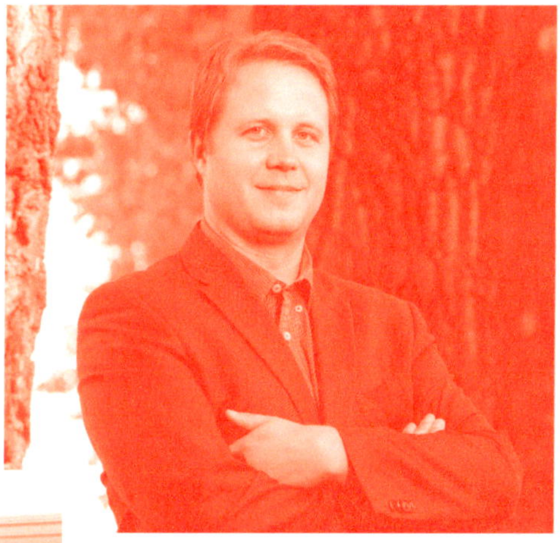

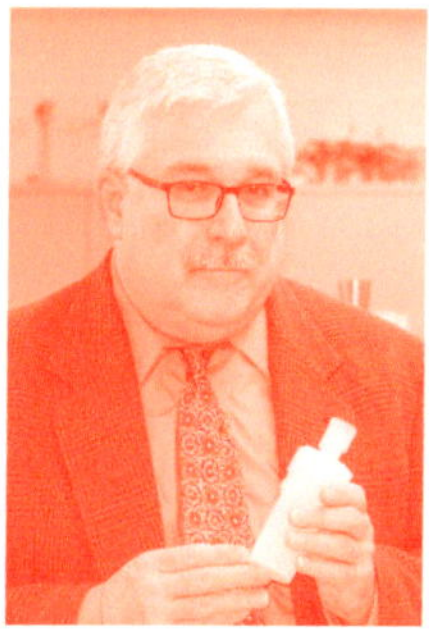

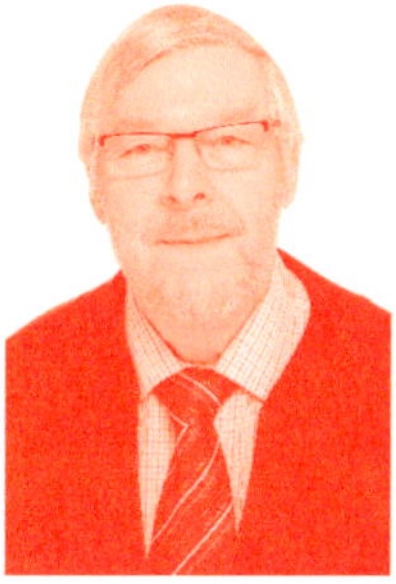

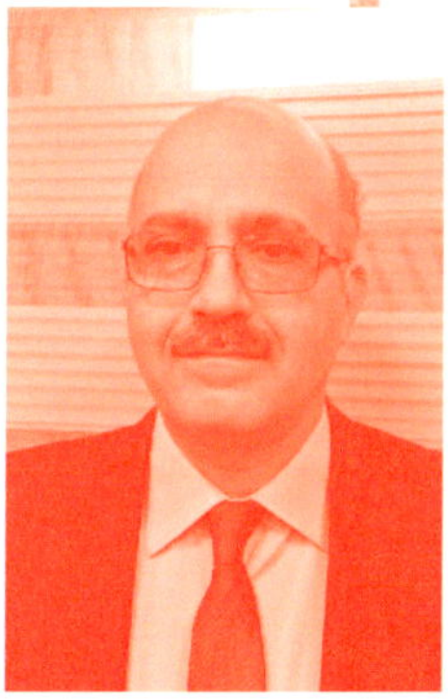

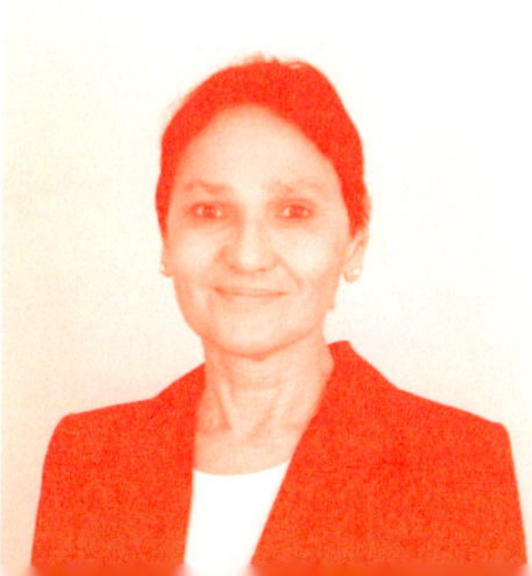

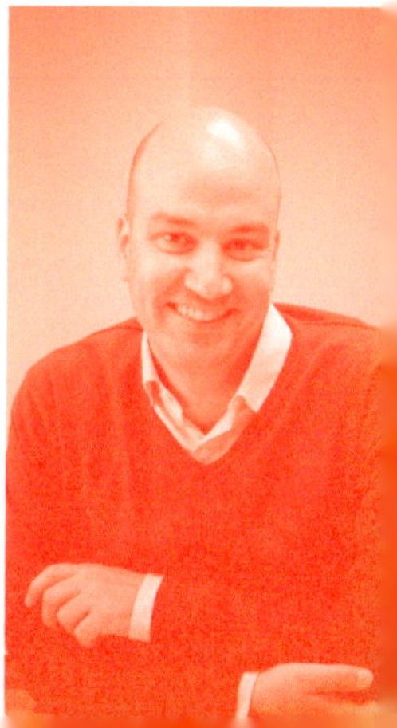

Organ Donation and Transplantation
http://dx.doi.org/10.5772/intechopen.87319
Edited by Vassil Mihaylov

Contributors
Željka Večerić-Haler, Neva Bezeljak, Ifeoma Ulasi, Chinwuba Ijoma, Ejikeme Arodiwe, Chimezie Okwuonu, Julius Okoye, Obinna Onodugo, Sani Alhassan, Ugochi Onu, Ngozi Ifebunandu, Uchenna Ijoma, Farzad Kakaei, Mehmet Nur Altınörs, Velislava Terzieva, Suresh Keshavamurthy, Vipin Dulam, Abul Kashem, Yoshiya Toyoda, Eros Leotta, Tatsuaki Tsuruyama, Omur Sayligil, Mesut Güvenbaş, Yordanka Uzunova, Radosvet Gornev, Lubomir Spassov

© The Editor(s) and the Author(s) 2021
The rights of the editor(s) and the author(s) have been asserted in accordance with the Copyright, Designs and Patents Act 1988. All rights to the book as a whole are reserved by INTECHOPEN LIMITED. The book as a whole (compilation) cannot be reproduced, distributed or used for commercial or non-commercial purposes without INTECHOPEN LIMITED's written permission. Enquiries concerning the use of the book should be directed to INTECHOPEN LIMITED rights and permissions department (permissions@intechopen.com).
Violations are liable to prosecution under the governing Copyright Law.

(cc) BY

Individual chapters of this publication are distributed under the terms of the Creative Commons Attribution 3.0 Unported License which permits commercial use, distribution and reproduction of the individual chapters, provided the original author(s) and source publication are appropriately acknowledged. If so indicated, certain images may not be included under the Creative Commons license. In such cases users will need to obtain permission from the license holder to reproduce the material. More details and guidelines concerning content reuse and adaptation can be found at http://www.intechopen.com/copyright-policy.html.

Notice
Statements and opinions expressed in the chapters are these of the individual contributors and not necessarily those of the editors or publisher. No responsibility is accepted for the accuracy of information contained in the published chapters. The publisher assumes no responsibility for any damage or injury to persons or property arising out of the use of any materials, instructions, methods or ideas contained in the book.

First published in London, United Kingdom, 2021 by IntechOpen
IntechOpen is the global imprint of INTECHOPEN LIMITED, registered in England and Wales, registration number: 11086078, 5 Princes Gate Court, London, SW7 2QJ, United Kingdom
Printed in Croatia

British Library Cataloguing-in-Publication Data
A catalogue record for this book is available from the British Library

Additional hard and PDF copies can be obtained from orders@intechopen.com

Organ Donation and Transplantation
Edited by Vassil Mihaylov
p. cm.
Print ISBN 978-1-83962-531-2
Online ISBN 978-1-83962-545-9
eBook (PDF) ISBN 978-1-83962-549-7

For EU product safety concerns:
IN TECH d.o.o., Prolaz Marije Krucifikse Kozulić 3, 51000 Rijeka, Croatia, info@intechopen.com or visit our website at intechopen.com.

We are IntechOpen, the world's leading publisher of Open Access books

Built by scientists, for scientists

5,200+
Open access books available

128,000+
International authors and editors

150M+
Downloads

156
Countries delivered to

Our authors are among the
Top 1%
most cited scientists

12.2%
Contributors from top 500 universities

WEB OF SCIENCE™

Selection of our books indexed in the Book Citation Index
in Web of Science™ Core Collection (BKCI)

Interested in publishing with us?
Contact book.department@intechopen.com

Numbers displayed above are based on latest data collected.
For more information visit www.intechopen.com

Meet the editor

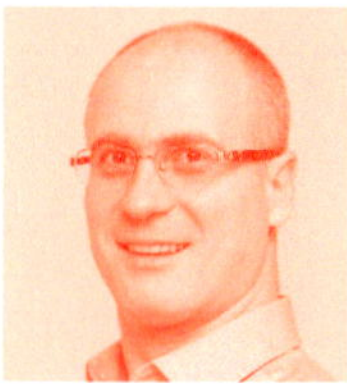

Dr. Vassil Mihaylov received his medical degree from the Medical University, Sofia, Bulgaria, and completed his general surgery residency at the Military Medical Academy, Sofia. He completed a transplant fellowship at Queen Elizabeth Hospital, Birmingham, UK, after which he returned to Sofia as a part of the HPB and transplant team at the Military Medical Academy. Dr. Mihaylov obtained his Ph.D. with a thesis on the surgical aspects of liver transplantation. He was appointed Associate Professor of Surgery in 2017. He has published more than 100 papers in peer-reviewed journals and has given many scientific presentations at international meetings. He is a Fellow of the American College of Surgeons and a member of several professional organizations including the Bulgarian Transplant Society, the European Society for Organ Transplantation (ESOT), International Liver Transplantation Society (ILTS), Society of Laparoscopic Surgeons, and International Hepato-Pancreato-Biliary Association (IHPBA). His clinical and research interests include hepatobiliary and pancreatic surgery, minimally invasive surgery, and liver transplantation.

Contents

Preface

The field of organ transplantation continues to evolve and is a highly effective therapy for patients with end-organ dysfunction (liver, kidney, pancreas, heart, lung) with a wide range of medical conditions. Improvement of perioperative care, surgical technique and immunosuppression in recent years has led to the transformation of organ transplantation into a safe and routine procedure with steadily improving results.

Organ donation plays a key role in the transplant process and corresponds to many fields of medical knowledge as well as social and ethical aspects. New advancements in surgery have allowed for more efficient and refined multi-organ procurements with minimal complications and decreased ischemic injury events. However, the increasing number of patients on transplant waiting lists and the limited donor pool have led to increased demand for new approaches, such as splitting organs, living donation and tissue engineering. In recent years, trends halve shifted towards marginal grafts, which are grafts from higher-risk donors.

Transplantation is a complex process that requires the effort and effective collaboration of a wide range of medical specialists (medical doctors, surgeons, anesthesiologists, psychologists, coordinators, etc.) and institutions. Good results are a function of the proper selection of donors and recipients. Further research will lead to a better understanding of the pathophysiology of the immune response and help scientists to develop more effective strategies for improving graft and patient survival.

Vassil Mihaylov, MD, PhD, FACS
Associate Professor,
HPB and Transplant surgery,
Military Medical Academy,
Sofia, Bulgaria

Section 1

Organ Donation

Chapter 1

Pathophysiological Changes and Systemic Inflammation in Brain Dead Organ Donors: Effect on Graft Quality

Neva Bezeljak and Željka Večerić-Haler

Abstract

Transplantation is the definitive treatment of end-stage organ disease. As the shortage of suitable organs poses its main limitation, the active management of potential organ donors becomes increasingly more important. The majority of solid organs are still obtained from donors after confirmed brain death. Brain death is the complete and irreversible cessation of all brain functions, and triggers a variety of severe pathophysiological changes in cardiovascular, hormonal and metabolic status that can result in organ damage. Moreover, brain death is associated with massive inflammatory response with a cytokine storm and complement activation that increases graft immunogenicity and adversely affects graft survival. Organs from brain-dead donors are more prone to graft dysfunction and rejection when compared to organs obtained from living donors. Brain death is thus believed to be an important risk factor influencing the quality of organs before procurement.

Keywords: inflammation brain death, pathophysiology brain death, systemic inflammation brain death, SIRS, donation after brain death, brain death, organ donation

1. Introduction

Transplantation is the definitive treatment for solid organ end-stage disease. The waiting list for organ transplant is growing rapidly and the available offer of suitable organs is not sufficient enough to satisfy the needs. Within the Eurotransplant region and worldwide, the majority of transplanted organs are obtained from deceased brain-dead donors [1].

It is well known that the results from kidney grafts retrieved from living donors (both related and unrelated to recipients) are far superior to those of deceased organ donors in terms of delayed graft function, acute rejection and graft survival [2–4]. As there is a significant difference between short- and long-term survival of kidneys from living and deceased donors, the focus has recently shifted from recipient to donor and the events occurring at the time of and after brain death.

Brain death is a catastrophic event resulting in severe systemic disturbance including haemodynamic instability, inflammatory, hormonal, metabolic and hematological disorders [5]. A limiting factor for better transplant outcome in a

 IntechOpen

potential organ donor is definitely activation of the immune system that starts early, during and immediately after brain death. For this reason, brain death has become one of the key factors believed to significantly impact transplant function and survival.

Early identification of potential donors is essential to establish timely and aggressive donor management so as to provide the quantity and quality of organs available for successful donation and transplantation. Unfortunately, no standardized guidelines for the management of brain-dead donors have been implemented to this moment [6]. Nevertheless, the main goal for successful organ donation is to normalize and maintain the physiological conditions, including haemodynamic stability, adequate oxygenation, and optimal fluid and electrolyte balance. Aggressive respiratory and haemodynamic monitoring is thus essential to prevent any unnecessary loss of organs [7].

2. Brain death-related pathophysiological systemic disorders

Brain death is a complete cessation of all brain functions, including the brain stem, when the etiology of brain dysfunction is known and considered irreversible. All reversible causes must be examined and excluded. The essential criteria for brain death, according to the American Academy of Neurology (AAN), are coma or unresponsiveness, absence of brain stem reflexes, and apnea. A patient determined to be brain dead is legally and clinically dead, and can be considered as organ donor in agreement with his own and his next of kin's choice [5]. Loss of central regulation leads to severe pathophysiological alterations in haemodynamics and the respiratory, inflammatory and endocrine systems [7, 8].

2.1 Cardiovascular changes

The increased intracranial pressure following cerebral trauma, infarction or hemorrhage causes increased arterial blood pressure as an attempt to restore adequate cerebral perfusion. In case this fails, ischemia of pons generates a reflex response, known as Cushing reflex, with bradycardia and hypertension. The ischemic damage then progresses through the entire brain and results in sympathetic stimulation and a catecholamine storm characterized by hypertension, tachycardia, and severe peripheral vasoconstriction. A more explosive increase of intracranial brain pressure correlates with a higher increase in catecholamine concentrations. Consequently, a significant reduction in blood flow prevails despite increased systemic perfusion pressure, and leads to visceral and myocardial ischemia [8, 9]. Observations in brain-dead donors show evidence of myocardial ischemia on echocardiographic exam [10, 11].

The initial phase of a catecholamine storm is followed by a loss of sympathetic tonus and profound vasodilation due to ischemia of the brain stem vasomotor nuclei. Many factors contribute to hypotension, including vasodilatation, catecholamine depletion, myocardial dysfunction, relative hypovolemia, and endocrine dysfunction. Hypoperfusion further deteriorates organ integrity and, together with a catecholamine explosion, leads to deleterious consequences for potential grafts if left untreated.

2.2 Pulmonary changes

Two main complications related to brain death-induced lung injury and dysfunction are neurogenic pulmonary edema and inflammatory acute lung injury.

Donors may also have specific pulmonary damage, including aspiration, atelectasis, contusion, chest trauma, or infection [12]. Volume overload after fluid resuscitation, also due to profound hypotension, increases the risk of pulmonary edema [8].

2.3 Endocrine system, stress and metabolic responses

Diabetes insipidus secondary to posterior pituitary infarction and lack of antidiuretic hormone results in electrolyte imbalance, hypovolemia, and circulatory instability. Thyroid hormonal changes and thyroid-stimulating hormone (TSH) levels show the typical picture of euthyroid sick syndrome. Temperature regulation in the hypothalamus is affected, manifesting with initial hyperthermia followed by hypothermia. Hypothermia, additionally worsened by peripheral vasodilatation, further aggravates acidosis and increases the risk for arrhythmias and cold-induced diuresis. Due to reduced insulin concentration and peripheral insulin resistance, hyperglycaemia is common [7, 12].

2.4 Hematological changes

Damaged brain tissue is a rich source of potent platelet-activating and procoagulant molecules, which often leads to disseminated intravascular coagulation. Hypothermia, acidosis and catecholamines all affect platelets function, further contributing to coagulopathy [13, 14].

3. Strategies to maintain pathophysiological changes in organ donors

The current recommendations and guidelines for the management of a potential organ donor in the intensive care unit (ICU) are based on pathophysiological reasoning and experience gained from general ICU management strategies, and not on evidence from randomized controlled trials (**Table 1**) [17]. The protection and optimization of organ functions in order to provide for a maximum number of quality organs that can be offered for donation is the essential goal of intensive care donor management. The purpose of this paper is not to describe the management of the donor in detail, as this was already summarized recently by Meyfroidt et al. [18]. A more simplified and easy-to-remember series of goals was established a decade ago, known as the "rule of 100": systolic arterial pressure > 100 mmHg, urine output >100 ml/hr., arterial partial pressure of oxygen (PaO2) >100 mmHg, hemoglobin concentration > 100 g/L, and blood sugar 100% normal [15].

4. Activation of inflammatory system

Aseptic necrosis of brain tissue leads to the release of numerous inflammatory mediators that trigger and support massive local and systemic inflammatory response driven by both the innate and adaptive immune systems. Catecholamine storm and hypotension with hypoperfusion of organs then contribute to the additional activation of immunologic pathways [19].

One of its harmful consequences is the activation of the cytokine system, polypeptide immunomodulatory molecules that participate in both immune responses and act on cell differentiation, proliferation and activity. Several cytokines have been found in brain tissue and cerebrospinal fluid after brain death. These cytokines are then delivered into circulation through a faulty blood–brain barrier, and continue to stimulate peripheral target cells and organs [20].

	Suggested approach
General care	Manage in ICU. Central and arterial line insertion and monitoring of central venous and arterial pressure. Cardiac output monitoring preferred. Nasogastric tube insertion. Foley's catheter insertion and measurement of urine output. Reduce heat loss and actively warm, if necessary, to maintain core temperature >35°C. Actively treat infections. Frequent airway suctioning. Maintain pneumatic compression device for preventing deep vein thrombosis. Eye protection. Ulcer prophylaxis. Broad spectrum antibiotics.
Respiratory	Use 'lung protective' ventilation (lowest possible plateau pressure, tidal volumes of 6 ml/kg of ideal body weight, and moderate positive end expiratory pressure [PEEP] of 5–10 cmH2O to achieve an oxygen saturation >92%). The respiratory passage must be kept clear of any obstruction with routine measures. Avoid the administration of excessive i.v. fluids.
Cardiovascular	Goals for the management of haemodynamic status in donors: (1) to maintain normovolaemia; (2) control blood pressure (BP); (3) optimize cardiac output and maintain perfusion pressure of all organs; and (4) to minimize the use of vasoactive agents. Review fluid balance and correct hypovolaemia. Monitor cardiac output to titrate fluids and inotropic/vasopressor drugs to intended goals. At present, there are no convincing studies or consensus to demonstrate that one vasopressor is superior to another, and different drugs (noradrenaline, adrenaline, vasopressin, dopamine, and/or dobutamine) are used, depending on local practices and protocols. High doses of catecholamines (e.g., norepinephrine >0.05 μg kg^{-1} min^{-1}) should be avoided, if possible.
Fluids and nutrition	Administer maintenance fluids, preferentially crystalloids with balanced salt content (lactated Ringer's solution and half-normal saline (0.45%) are most frequently used) to avoid hypernatremia. Avoid volume overload. Correct electrolyte abnormalities to normal values. Blood glucose target concentrations 4–8 mmol/ litre. A solution of 0.9% normal saline may cause hyperchloremic acidosis, which increases renal vascular resistance. Colloids, such as hydroxyethyl starches, need to be avoided in organ donors, as they can damage renal epithelial cells and cause early graft dysfunction in the transplanted kidneys. Albumin solutions can be used to reduce the amount of fluid volume administered.
Blood and coagulation	Consider the need for transfusion. The target is to maintain the hematocrit above 30%. Maintain thromboprophylaxis, as there is a high incidence of embolisms. Coagulopathy should be treated promptly with management, including the administration of red blood cells, clotting factors, and platelets.
Systemic effects	Corticosteroids. The main purpose of using corticosteroids is not to treat adrenocortical failure, but rather to attenuate the immune responses and reduce the catecholamine requirement for maintaining BP. Methylprednisolone 15 mg kg^{-1} bolus is recommended immediately after brain death is confirmed. Triiodothyronine. Routine replacement of thyroid hormones is not recommended for all organ donors, but only if impaired cardiac performance is documented despite overall good general management and in case of patients with true hypothyroidism. Insulin. Hyperglycemia is closely associated with reduced host immune responses that result in an increased risk of infection, worsening of renal function in renal transplant recipients, as well as osmotic diuresis [16]. Hyperglycemic organ donor patients should be treated according to the local institutional guidelines used for other critically ill patients. Anti-diuretic hormone. If the patient develops diabetes insipidus, the condition can be treated by the replacement of fluid with adequate crystalloid solutions. However, if hypotension persists despite adequate volume resuscitation in the absence of other causes, treatment with vasopressin or DDAVP should be considered.

DDAVP, 1-deamino-8-D-arginine-vasopressin; PEEP, positive end-expiratory pressure.

Table 1.
Summary of the principles of donor management (adapted from Anwar et al. [7] and McKeown et al. [15]).

The up-regulated expression of cell adhesion molecules (CAMs), including selectines, vascular (VCAM-1) and intracellular CAMs (ICAM-1) on the endothelium of potential grafts plays a critical role in numerous inflammatory processes. One of their tasks is the recruitment of circulating monocytes, macrophages and polymorphonuclear leukocytes as shown in organ biopsies after organ retrieval [12, 16, 21, 22]. Therefore, unsurprisingly, increased levels of CAMs have been associated with increased mortality in transplant recipients [16].

The activation of leukocyte populations in peripheral organs further maintains an inflammatory environment by expressing CAMs and releasing proinflammatory substances, among others, tumor necrosis factor alpha (TNF-α) and interferon gamma (IFN-γ) [16]. Especially IFN-γ induces the expression of major histocompatibility complex (MHC) classes I and II on graft cells, which potentiate the immunogenicity of organs via the T-cell recognition process. The activated organs provoke a host immune system after engraftment, resulting in severe acute or chronic rejection [23].

Complement activation has already been demonstrated in ischemia–reperfusion injury and rejection. Fragments of complement activation products have been measured in plasma and organ biopsies. Their values were higher compared to living donors [24–26].

4.1 Cytokines implicated in brain death

Increased blood levels of several cytokines, such as TNF-α, interleukin (IL)-6, IL-8, IL-1β, and IL-2R, have been observed after brain death [27, 28]. Cytokines derive mostly from T-cells and are classified into different groups according to their main function and T helper (Th) cell subtypes to which they are related.

The Th1-cell related cytokines are TNF-α, IL-1, IL-2, IL-12 and IFN-γ [29, 30]. They act early in the inflammatory cascade and stimulate and support the inflammation by mediating between different inflammatory pathways; they activate endothelial cells and cellular adhesion molecules, and contribute to T-cell maturation.

The Th2-cell-related cytokines IL-4, IL-5, IL-10 and IL-13 are not as significant and are considered to be anti-inflammatory when related to brain death and the early transplant period [19, 31, 32].

One of the most heavily implicated cytokines in brain death is IL-6, a member of Th-17 cell related mediators [33, 34]. Increased concentrations of IL-6 have been demonstrated both in plasma and organs of brain-dead donors, including the kidneys, lungs, liver and heart [34–36]. Higher values of IL - 6 are associated with worse transplantation outcomes and poorer survival of recipients [33, 37].

A significant increase in IL-8 values in the bronchoalveolar lavage fluid from brain-dead lung donors has been demonstrated and correlates with early graft dysfunction after lung transplant [38]. In addition, elevated IL-6 gene expression was observed in the preimplantation biopsies of patients who died within 30 days after lung transplant [39]. Furthermore, the levels of IL-1β and TNF-α were significantly higher in donor lungs rejected for transplantation compared to transplanted lungs [40]. The values of IL-6 and TNF-α in the myocardium of dysfunctional discarded donor hearts were higher than in transplanted donor hearts [41].

4.2 Role of complement

The complement cascade is an important part of the innate immune system and transplantation process. Activation of either the classic, alternative or lectin pathway of the complement system leads to the formation of a common terminal cell lytic complex or C5b-9, also known as membrane attack complex (MAC). MAC induces complement-mediated lysis of cells. Proteolytic complement fragments such as C5a, C3a and, to a lesser extent, C4a, further induce acute inflammation by activating mast cells, neutrophils and endothelial cells.

Studies have shown that all three pathway types are involved in systemic inflammation secondary to brain death [24]. Complement activation products have the ability to produce proinflammatory substances, including cytokines, and act as chemotactic factors for leukocytes.

In deceased brain donors, the increased complement plasma levels of C5b9 were higher than in the plasma of living organ donors. Higher levels of C5b9 in deceased brain-dead and deceased cardiac-dead donors were associated with worse tissue damage, a higher rate of acute and chronic rejection, and inferior function after transplantation [25].

Complement activation also results in the release of anaphylatoxins C3a and C5a, potent activators of T-cells. Brain-dead organ donors had higher values of C5a in plasma compared to living donors [26].

5. Inflammation limiting strategies

5.1 Inflammation limiting strategies in organ donors

The use of methylprednisolone, alone or as part of hormonal replacement, reduces the immunological activation observed after brain death in terms of decreasing cytokine production and preventing alterations induced by proinflammatory mediators [36, 42]. In a prospective randomized study, reduced serum and graft cytokine expression and improved graft function in human liver transplantation was found/reported after methylprednisolone administration [42]. Inflammation in the heart and kidneys is also reduced. The reduction in cytokine activation is almost comparable to the levels seen in living donor transplantation [36]. Methylprednisolone use is associated with increased organ retrieval and improved short- and long-term outcome for most transplanted organs [12].

Numerous other agents and approaches are currently under investigation as part of organ protection and preservation strategies.

Among such strategies, active removal of cytokines by haemoadsorption was shown to be feasible, leading to at least a moderate fall in cytokine concentration in circulation, attenuating the inflammatory response associated with brain death [9].

Although no RCTs in humans currently exist, animal models have also demonstrated a reduced inflammatory response and improved oxygenation when using noradrenaline [43, 44].

Since glucagon-like peptide-1 (GLP1) analogues were shown to possess interesting cytoprotective effects in different liver and pancreatic disease models, these molecules were also tested in experimental transplantation models. Treatment with the GLP1 analogue exendin-4 (Ex-4) relieved brain dead-induced liver [45], renal [46] and pancreatic islet injury [47] through alleviation of inflammation and oxidative stress.

After single administration of antithymocyte globulin (ATG) to brain-dead mice, the inflammatory reaction in the myocardium showed a significant reduction in IL-2 expression and the reduction of IL-6 deposition in media cells in ATG-treated specimens compared to controls [48].

Targeting complement activation after the induction of brain death also reduced renal inflammation and improved renal function before transplantation in animal models [49]. Recently, a study by Jager et al. [50]. has shown that experimental donor rat pre-treatment with anti-FB preserved renal function reduced renal damage and inflammation prior to transplantation. Seemingly, high-dose C1-INH treatment of brain-dead rat donors resulted in significantly lower renal gene expression and serum levels of IL-6, which reflected with improved renal function and reduced renal injury [51].

Traumatic brain injury and other inflammatory conditions are currently being treated in preclinical and clinical trials by a number of cellular therapies, among which mesenchymal stem cells (MSC) are of greatest interest due to their widespread usage and ease to isolate and culture [52, 53].

Therefore, strategies targeting cytokine and complement activation in human brain-dead donors pose as a new and promising opportunity to improve organ quantity and quality for successful organ donation and transplantation outcome.

5.2 Inflammation limiting strategies to preserve procured organs

After procurement, organs are further exposed to injury due to removal from their physiological conditions. Hypoxic injury has a detrimental effect on organ structure and function, and adds to increased immunogenicity. Prolonged ischemia, cold or warm, is a risk factor for early graft dysfunction and worse long-term outcomes. The duration and type (warm or cold) of ischemia time may also directly influence cytokine production [19]. Significant cytokine gene expression has otherwise already occurred directly after brain death. Namely, the cytokine gene expression before transplantation was shown to be even higher than during the period of acute rejection [35]. A strong association was recently identified between cold ischemia time and the levels of IL-1 and IL-8 in human liver transplants. Warm ischemia time also correlated with IL-6 and IL-10 in the same study [54].

Successful preservation strategies are key to minimize ischemic damage and the effect of reperfusion with associated increased immunogenicity after organ implantation. The current accepted standard for most solid organs is static cold storage (SCS), where the solid organ is stored on ice after removal from the donor, and then removed from the ice box at the time of implantation. However, novel technologies enable perfusion of the donated organ during the transport phase or at the recipient centre, with the option to use a variety of temperatures and different perfusates. Machine perfusion systems (hypothermic, normothermic, oxygen persufflation) represent dynamic preservational methods.

Hypothermic preservation strategies are now widely used to decrease inflammation, depress the metabolic rate of cells, and reduce the effects of ischemia [55, 56]. In the largest meta-analysis performed so far [57], hypothermic machine perfusion (HMP) was superior to SCS in deceased donor kidney transplantation (this was true for both DBD and DCD kidneys). The incidence of delayed graft function in kidneys from deceased brain donors was much lower in the group with hypothermic perfusion. Additionally, reports of economic analysis suggested that HMP can lead to cost savings in both North American and European settings.

Since very low temperatures can also have harmful repercussions on organs in terms of cytokine and reactive oxygen production [58], over the last two decades several research groups have examined the effects of increasing the temperature of machine perfusion to near-normothermic temperatures (20–33°C). Near-normothermic preservation is particularly applicable for organs of marginal donors or donors after cardiac death. In these cases, due to prolonged warm ischemia times, organ viability is negatively impacted by the subsequent cold preservation. Hence, normothermic perfusion may enhance preservation and transplantation outcomes and reduce the risk of non-functional organs [59].

6. Conclusion

Brain-dead organ donors represent the major source of organs for organ transplantation. The path from a brain-dead potential donor to a favorable graft and recipient outcome is long, and can have a cardinal impact on the quality of transplanted organs. Brain death-related systemic changes can damage the organs to the point where donation is not possible. Severe systemic inflammatory response enhances graft immunogenicity and affects graft survival and transplant outcome. Thus, immunomodulatory agents can become pivotal in donor procurement and preservation in future.

Conflict of interest

The authors declare no conflict of interest.

Author details

Neva Bezeljak[1] and Željka Večerić-Haler[1,2]*

1 Department of Nephrology, University Medical Centre Ljubljana, Slovenia

2 Medical Faculty, University of Ljubljana, Slovenia

*Address all correspondence to: zeljka.vecerichaler@kclj.si

IntechOpen

© 2020 The Author(s). Licensee IntechOpen. This chapter is distributed under the terms of the Creative Commons Attribution License (http://creativecommons.org/licenses/by/3.0), which permits unrestricted use, distribution, and reproduction in any medium, provided the original work is properly cited.

References

[1] *Annual Report 2019: infographic with highlights*. Available from: https://www.eurotransplant.org/statistics/annual-report/.

[2] Nemati, E., et al., *Does kidney transplantation with deceased or living donor affect graft survival?* Nephrourol Mon, 2014. **6**(4): p. e12182.

[3] Nijboer, W.N., et al., *Effect of brain death on gene expression and tissue activation in human donor kidneys.* Transplantation, 2004. **78**(7): p. 978-86.

[4] Terasaki, P.I., et al., *High survival rates of kidney transplants from spousal and living unrelated donors.* N Engl J Med, 1995. **333**(6): p. 333-6.

[5] Wijdicks, E.F., et al., *Evidence-based guideline update: determining brain death in adults: report of the Quality Standards Subcommittee of the American Academy of Neurology.* Neurology, 2010. **74**(23): p. 1911-8.

[6] Hahnenkamp, K., et al., *Organ-Protective Intensive Care in Organ Donors.* Dtsch Arztebl Int, 2016. **113**(33-34): p. 552-8.

[7] Anwar, A. and J.M. Lee, *Medical Management of Brain-Dead Organ Donors.* Acute Crit Care, 2019. **34**(1): p. 14-29.

[8] Kumar, L., *Brain death and care of the organ donor.* J Anaesthesiol Clin Pharmacol, 2016. **32**(2): p. 146-52.

[9] Kellum, J.A., et al., *Feasibility study of cytokine removal by hemoadsorption in brain-dead humans.* Crit Care Med, 2008. **36**(1): p. 268-72.

[10] Dujardin, K.S., et al., *Myocardial dysfunction associated with brain death: clinical, echocardiographic, and pathologic features.* J Heart Lung Transplant, 2001. **20**(3): p. 350-7.

[11] Venkateswaran, R.V., et al., *Echocardiography in the potential heart donor.* Transplantation, 2010. **89**(7): p. 894-901.

[12] Bugge, J.F., *Brain death and its implications for management of the potential organ donor.* Acta Anaesthesiol Scand, 2009. **53**(10): p. 1239-50.

[13] Talving, P., et al., *Coagulopathy in severe traumatic brain injury: a prospective study.* J Trauma, 2009. **66**(1): p. 55-61; discussion 61-2.

[14] Zhang, J., et al., *Traumatic brain injury-associated coagulopathy.* J Neurotrauma, 2012. **29**(17): p. 2597-605.

[15] McKeown, D.W., R.S. Bonser, and J.A. Kellum, *Management of the heartbeating brain-dead organ donor.* Br J Anaesth, 2012. **108 Suppl 1**: p. i96-107.

[16] Connolly, G.M., et al., *Elevated soluble cellular adhesion molecules are associated with increased mortality in a prospective cohort of renal transplant recipients.* BMC Nephrol, 2011. **12**: p. 23.

[17] Kotloff, R.M., et al., *Management of the Potential Organ Donor in the ICU: Society of Critical Care Medicine/American College of Chest Physicians/Association of Organ Procurement Organizations Consensus Statement.* Crit Care Med, 2015. **43**(6): p. 1291-325.

[18] Meyfroidt, G., et al., *Management of the brain-dead donor in the ICU: general and specific therapy to improve transplantable organ quality.* Intensive Care Med, 2019. **45**(3): p. 343-353.

[19] Watts, R.P., O. Thom, and J.F. Fraser, *Inflammatory signalling associated with brain dead organ donation: from brain injury to brain stem death and posttransplant ischaemia reperfusion*

injury. J Transplant, 2013. **2013**: p. 521369.

[20] Kostulas, N., et al., *Increased IL-1beta, IL-8, and IL-17 mRNA expression in blood mononuclear cells observed in a prospective ischemic stroke study.* Stroke, 1999. **30**(10): p. 2174-9.

[21] Koo, D.D., et al., *Cadaver versus living donor kidneys: impact of donor factors on antigen induction before transplantation.* Kidney Int, 1999. **56**(4): p. 1551-9.

[22] van Der Hoeven, J.A., et al., *Effects of brain death and hemodynamic status on function and immunologic activation of the potential donor liver in the rat.* Ann Surg, 2000. **232**(6): p. 804-13.

[23] Pratschke, J., et al., *Accelerated rejection of renal allografts from brain-dead donors.* Ann Surg, 2000. **232**(2): p. 263-71.

[24] Damman, J., et al., *Hypoxia and Complement-and-Coagulation Pathways in the Deceased Organ Donor as the Major Target for Intervention to Improve Renal Allograft Outcome.* Transplantation, 2015. **99**(6): p. 1293-300.

[25] Damman, J., et al., *Systemic complement activation in deceased donors is associated with acute rejection after renal transplantation in the recipient.* Transplantation, 2011. **92**(2): p. 163-9.

[26] van Werkhoven, M.B., et al., *Complement mediated renal inflammation induced by donor brain death: role of renal C5a-C5aR interaction.* Am J Transplant, 2013. **13**(4): p. 875-882.

[27] Skrabal, C.A., et al., *Organ-specific regulation of pro-inflammatory molecules in heart, lung, and kidney following brain death.* J Surg Res, 2005. **123**(1): p. 118-25.

[28] Stangl, M., et al., *Influence of brain death on cytokine release in organ donors and renal transplants.* Transplant Proc, 2001. **33**(1-2): p. 1284-5.

[29] Huss, D.J., et al., *TGF-beta enhances effector Th1 cell activation but promotes self-regulation via IL-10.* J Immunol, 2010. **184**(10): p. 5628-36.

[30] Itoh, S., et al., *Interleukin-17 accelerates allograft rejection by suppressing regulatory T cell expansion.* Circulation, 2011. **124**(11 Suppl): p. S187-96.

[31] Deknuydt, F., et al., *IL-1beta and IL-2 convert human Treg into T(H)17 cells.* Clin Immunol, 2009. **131**(2): p. 298-307.

[32] Xiong, X., et al., *Increased brain injury and worsened neurological outcome in interleukin-4 knockout mice after transient focal cerebral ischemia.* Stroke, 2011. **42**(7): p. 2026-32.

[33] Murugan, R., et al., *Increased plasma interleukin-6 in donors is associated with lower recipient hospital-free survival after cadaveric organ transplantation.* Crit Care Med, 2008. **36**(6): p. 1810-6.

[34] Plenz, G., et al., *The interleukin-6/interleukin-6-receptor system is activated in donor hearts.* J Am Coll Cardiol, 2002. **39**(9): p. 1508-12.

[35] Kaminska, D., et al., *Cytokine gene expression in kidney allograft biopsies after donor brain death and ischemia-reperfusion injury using in situ reverse-transcription polymerase chain reaction analysis.* Transplantation, 2007. **84**(9): p. 1118-24.

[36] Kuecuek, O., et al., *Significant reduction of proinflammatory cytokines by treatment of the brain-dead donor.* Transplant Proc, 2005. **37**(1): p. 387-8.

[37] Murugan, R., et al., *Preload responsiveness is associated with increased interleukin-6 and lower organ yield from*

brain-dead donors. Crit Care Med, 2009. **37**(8): p. 2387-93.

[38] Fisher, A.J., et al., *Elevated levels of interleukin-8 in donor lungs is associated with early graft failure after lung transplantation.* Am J Respir Crit Care Med, 2001. **163**(1): p. 259-65.

[39] Kaneda, H., et al., *Pre-implantation multiple cytokine mRNA expression analysis of donor lung grafts predicts survival after lung transplantation in humans.* Am J Transplant, 2006. **6**(3): p. 544-51.

[40] Cypel, M., et al., *Increased levels of interleukin-1beta and tumor necrosis factor-alpha in donor lungs rejected for transplantation.* J Heart Lung Transplant, 2011. **30**(4): p. 452-9.

[41] Birks, E.J., et al., *Elevated tumor necrosis factor-alpha and interleukin-6 in myocardium and serum of malfunctioning donor hearts.* Circulation, 2000. **102**(19 Suppl 3): p. III352-8.

[42] Kotsch, K., et al., *Methylprednisolone therapy in deceased donors reduces inflammation in the donor liver and improves outcome after liver transplantation: a prospective randomized controlled trial.* Ann Surg, 2008. **248**(6): p. 1042-50.

[43] Avlonitis, V.S., et al., *Early hemodynamic injury during donor brain death determines the severity of primary graft dysfunction after lung transplantation.* Am J Transplant, 2007. 7(1): p. 83-90.

[44] Avlonitis, V.S., et al., *The hemodynamic mechanisms of lung injury and systemic inflammatory response following brain death in the transplant donor.* Am J Transplant, 2005. **5**(4 Pt 1): p. 684-93.

[45] Carlessi, R., et al., *Exendin-4 attenuates brain death-induced liver damage in the rat.* Liver Transpl, 2015. **21**(11): p. 1410-8.

[46] Lemos, N.E., et al., *Renal effects of exendin-4 in an animal model of brain death.* Mol Biol Rep, 2019. **46**(2): p. 2197-2207.

[47] Carlessi, R., et al., *Exendin-4 protects rat islets against loss of viability and function induced by brain death.* Mol Cell Endocrinol, 2015. **412**: p. 239-50.

[48] Kremer, J., et al., *Influence of antithymocyte globulin treatment of brain-dead organ donor on inflammatory response in cardiac grafts: an experimental study in mice.* Transpl Int, 2016. **29**(12): p. 1329-1336.

[49] Fremeaux-Bacchi, V. and C.M. Legendre, *The emerging role of complement inhibitors in transplantation.* Kidney Int, 2015. **88**(5): p. 967-73.

[50] Jager, N.M., et al., *Blocking Complement Factor B Activation Reduces Renal Injury and Inflammation in a Rat Brain Death Model.* Front Immunol, 2019. **10**: p. 2528.

[51] Poppelaars, F., et al., *C1-Inhibitor Treatment Decreases Renal Injury in an Established Brain-Dead Rat Model.* Transplantation, 2018. **102**(1): p. 79-87.

[52] Kota, D.J., et al., *Prostaglandin E2 Indicates Therapeutic Efficacy of Mesenchymal Stem Cells in Experimental Traumatic Brain Injury.* Stem Cells, 2017. **35**(5): p. 1416-1430.

[53] Pacienza, N., et al., *Mesenchymal Stem Cell Therapy Facilitates Donor Lung Preservation by Reducing Oxidative Damage during Ischemia.* Stem Cells Int, 2019. **2019**: p. 8089215.

[54] Duran, J.A., et al., *Variation in the levels of inflammatory cytokines depending on ischemic time: effects on respiratory variables.* Transplant Proc, 2009. **41**(3): p. 980-2.

[55] Hosgood, S.A., et al., *Hypothermic machine perfusion after static cold storage does not improve the preservation condition in an experimental porcine kidney model.* Br J Surg, 2011. **98**(7): p. 943-50.

[56] Moers, C., et al., *Machine perfusion or cold storage in deceased-donor kidney transplantation.* N Engl J Med, 2009. **360**(1): p. 7-19.

[57] Tingle, S.J., et al., *Machine perfusion preservation versus static cold storage for deceased donor kidney transplantation.* Cochrane Database Syst Rev, 2019. **3**: p. CD011671.

[58] Guibert, E.E., et al., *Organ Preservation: Current Concepts and New Strategies for the Next Decade.* Transfus Med Hemother, 2011. **38**(2): p. 125-142.

[59] Salehi, S., K. Tran, and W.L. Grayson, *Advances in Perfusion Systems for Solid Organ Preservation.* Yale J Biol Med, 2018. **91**(3): p. 301-312.

Chapter 2

Organ Donation and Transplantation in Sub-Saharan Africa: Opportunities and Challenges

Ifeoma Ulasi, Chinwuba Ijoma, Ngozi Ifebunandu, Ejikeme Arodiwe, Uchenna Ijoma, Julius Okoye, Ugochi Onu, Chimezie Okwuonu, Sani Alhassan and Obinna Onodugo

Abstract

Sub-Saharan Africa (SSA), occupying about 80% of the African continent is a heterogeneous region with estimated population of 1.1 billion people in 47 countries. Most belong to the low resource countries (LRCs). The high prevalence of end-organ diseases of kidney, liver, lung and heart makes provision of organ donation and transplantation necessary. Although kidney and heart transplantations were performed in South Africa in the 1960s, transplant activity in SSA lags behind the developed world. Peculiar challenges militating against successful development of transplant programmes include high cost of treatment, low GDP of most countries, inadequate infrastructural and institutional support, absence of subsidy, poor knowledge of the disease condition, poor accessibility to healthcare facilities, religious and trado-cultural practices. Many people in the region patronize alternative healthcare as first choice. Opportunities that if harnessed may alter the unfavorable landscape are: implementation of the 2007 WHO Regional Consultation recommendations for establishment of national legal framework and self-sufficient organ donation/transplantation in each country and adoption of their 2020 proposed actions for organ/transplantation for member states, national registries with sharing of data with GODT, prevention of transplant commercialization and tourism. Additionally, adapting some aspects of proven successful models in LRCs will improve transplantation programmes in SSA.

Keywords: opportunities, challenges, low resource countries, end organ diseases/failure, transplant models

1. Introduction and overview

1.1 Background

Many diseases especially non-communicable diseases (NCDs) culminate in end-stage organ failures; the preferred treatment for most end-stage organ diseases is transplantation. Transplantation programme is a complex healthcare service

IntechOpen

which entails huge costs and requires highly skilled health professionals, complex infrastructure and equipment, and well-articulated legal frameworks to enable its operationalization [1]. The need for appropriate interventions for organ failures in sub-Saharan Africa (SSA) is underscored by the high prevalence of end-organ diseases such as chronic kidney disease (CKD), chronic liver disease (CLD), chronic lung and heart diseases (interstitial lung disease, cystic fibrosis, cardiomyopathies and chronic rheumatic heart diseases) which cause increased morbidity and mortality. For example, Kaze *et al* [2] in a systematic review of prevalence studies on CKD in SSA documented the highest prevalence in West Africa 19.8%, Central Africa 16%, East Africa 14.4%, and Southern Africa 10.4%.

Globally, beside organs, tissues and cells (bone marrow cornea, etc.) are also transplanted. However, in SSA, apart from South Africa which also does liver and heart transplantation, the common organ transplanted is the kidney [3]. Though outcomes for transplantation have improved over the years due to better surgical techniques including minimal access surgeries, newer and better immunosuppressive medications, innovations in organ donation; improvement in transplant services is not apparent in SSA. Organ transplantation remains largely inaccessible and unaffordable to this population.

Sub-Saharan Africa has a disproportionate burden of communicable diseases (CDs) and NCDs compared to other world regions [4]. Currently, NCDs are responsible for a large and increasing burden of death and disability in the region. World Health Organization (WHO) in 2018, documented that NCDs killed 41 million people per year accounting for 71% of the global deaths [5]. The ages most affected were 30 to 69 years age-group, belonging to the productive workforce of any population. People from low income countries (LICs) and lower-middle income countries (LMICs) accounted for most of these deaths approximating over 85%. Four of the five commonly quoted diseases i.e. the "Big Five" (cardiovascular diseases, cancers, respiratory diseases, diabetes mellitus (DM) and mental illness) that account for most NCD deaths are drivers of CKD. Several risk factors with multiplier effect on NCDs are tobacco use, physical inactivity, harmful use of alcohol and unhealthy diets. Communicable diseases, though less common in high income countries (HICs) and upper-middle income countries (UMICs) are still prevalent in LICs and LMICs prompting WHO to highlight the double burden of diseases in these regions [6]. Both CDs and NCDs culminate in end-organ disease underscoring the high prevalence of end-organ failures, disabilities and deaths in SSA (see **Figure 1**). Unfortunately, most countries in this region lack resources to cope.

1.2 Prevalence of end-organ diseases

1.2.1 End-stage kidney disease (ESKD)

In 2014, Stanifer *et al* [7], in a systematic review and meta-analysis of 21 studies in SSA documented an overall CKD prevalence of 13·9%. According to the Institute for Health Metrics and Evaluation (IHME) data, CKD and DM were the 14th cause of death in SSA in 1990 but worsened to 11th by 2017 (see **Figure 1**). Hypertension and DM constitute the main NCDs that cause CKD globally [8]. In many low resource countries (LRCs), chronic glomerulonephritis and interstitial nephritis assume significance because of the pervading and persisting high prevalence of CDs (mainly bacterial, parasitic, and viral infections) [9]. Human Immunodeficiency virus (HIV) infection which continues to plague SSA, albeit better controlled, is a key driver of kidney disease. Of the 38 million people living with HIV globally, more than 25 million live in this region [10, 11]. The recent pandemic of COVID-19 infection which has adverse acute effects on the kidney has probable

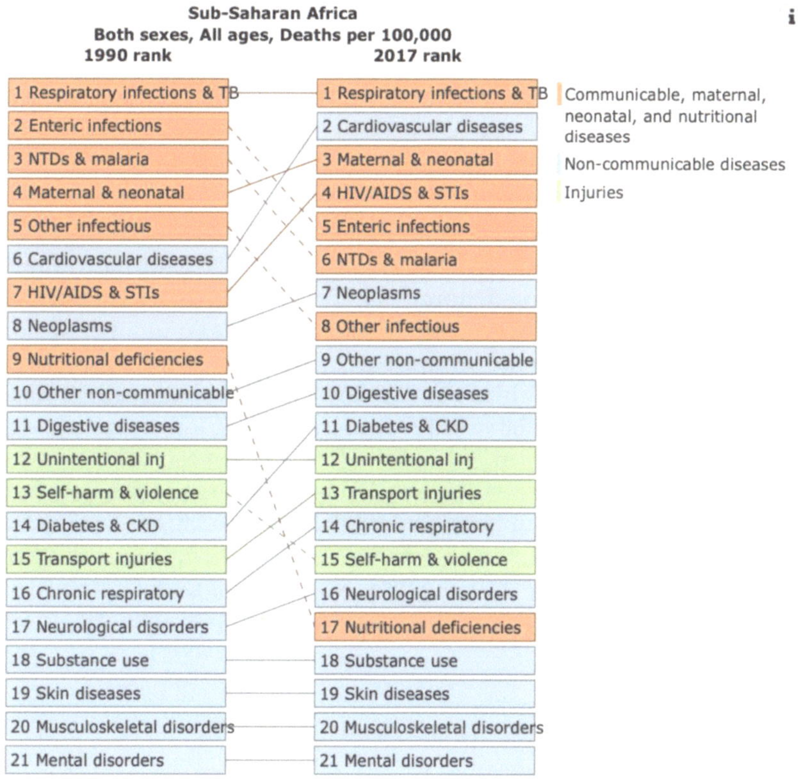

Figure 1.
Causes of deaths in sub Saharan Afirca 1990 and 2017 [from Institute for Health Metrics and Evaluation (IHME) data].

unknown long-term sequelae [12]. Both CDs and NCDs fuel the high and increasing prevalence of CKD in LRCs. Without renal registries in many LRCs, there is poor documentation of data on kidney diseases.

1.2.2 Other end-organ diseases

Viral hepatitis is prevalent in Africa with high endemicity of Hepatitis B Virus (HBV) in SSA and Hepatitis C virus (HCV) in North Africa. Africa has approximately 60–100 million of the world's 257 million viral hepatitis infections [13]. The WHO noted that between 1980 and 2010, cirrhosis-related deaths doubled in the region. The increasing burden of obesity and DM leading to non-alcoholic fatty liver disease contributes to high prevalence of CLD and end-stage liver disease (ESLD). Up to 40% of patients with chronic hepatitis may progress to liver cirrhosis and/or liver cancer [14] and without liver transplantation mortality is estimated at about 15% in one year [15]. All patients with ESLD will invariably require liver transplantation; however, liver transplants are uncommon in SSA.

There is scant information on prevalence of other end organ failures such as heart, lung, and small bowel requiring organ transplantation in SSA.

1.3 Prevalence of transplantation

The WHO in collaboration with the Organización Nacional de Trasplantes of Spain set up the Global Observatory on Donation and Transplantation (GODT) with the mandate to document the distribution of organ transplantation programmes in the countries that report their data to the Observatory and to evaluate the access of transplantation activities worldwide [16]. Upon subsequent request of the World Health Assembly (Resolutions WHA57.18 and 63.22) that global data on the practices, safety, quality, efficacy, epidemiology and ethical issues of allogeneic transplantation be collected and documented, the GODT was inaugurated in 2007 [16]. This database has ensured provision of transparent and equitable monitoring of national transplant systems.

Currently, according to the GODT database, [17], 139,024 solid organ transplants were reported globally in 2017: 90,306 kidney (36% from living donors), 32,348 liver (19.0% from living donors), 7881 heart, 6084 lung, 2243 pancreas and 162 small bowel transplants. Africa contributes the least number of transplant activity per continent and SSA the least number per WHO World region (**Tables 1** and **2**; **Figure 2**). **Tables 1** and **2** show data from 2016 GODT Report.

Kidney transplants are available in 102 countries; living kidney transplants in 98 countries and deceased donors in 76 countries [16]. Sixteen countries representing 6.6% of the global population perform only living donor kidney transplants. In SSA, a handful of countries carry out transplantation: South Africa, Sudan, Seychelles, Ivory Coast, Namibia, Nigeria, Kenya, Ghana, Tanzania, Mauritius, Ethiopia but only five countries (Ethiopia (0.34 pmp), Kenya (1.51 pmp), Nigeria (0.47 pmp), South Africa (6.81 pmp) and Sudan (6.58 pmp)) report their data to GODT (**Figure 2**).

1.4 Characteristics of SSA

1.4.1 Geography and demography

Sub-Saharan Africa is heterogeneous and has a population estimated at 1.1billion [18]. It is projected that countries in this region would account for more than half of the world's growth by 2050 [19]. This geographical region fully or partially located south of the Sahara Desert occupies an area of about 24 million Km^2 (**Figure 3**). It is made up of 47 countries divided into 4 WHO sub-regions. Most countries in this region belong to the LICs and LMICs according to World Bank Classification of economies and are also described as LRCs. Africa is the second largest and second most populous continent; SSA occupies about 80% of the continent [20]. Although the economic growth in Africa has been remarkable in recent years, the gap between the rich and poor is wide and many people still do not have access to basic amenities such as potable water, good sanitation and basic health services [20].

Region	Countries N	Countries with data N (%)	Population millions	Population with data millions (%)
AFR	46	10 (21.7)	1139.1	506.6 (44.5)
AMR	35	21 (60.0)	986.5	968.5 (98.2)
EMR	22	15 (68.2)	656.1	535 (81.5)
EUR	53	49 (92.5)	909.7	904.2 (99.4)
SEAR	11	5 (45.5)	1928.4	1408.8 (73.1)
WPR	27	11 (40.7)	1847.7	1815.3 (98.3)
Total	**194**	**111 (57.2)**	**7467.5**	**6138.4 (82.2)**

Table 1.
Proportion of countries and population covered by the GODT database in the WHO regions. Year 2015 [17].

	Africa Region (AFR)	America Region (AMR)	Eastern Mediterranean Region (EMR)	Europe (EUR)	South East Asia Region (SEAR)	Western Pacific Region (WPR)
Kidney	488 (1.0)	31,859 (32.9)	6127 (11.5)	26,131 (28.9)	7202 (5.1)	12,540 (6.9)
Liver	67 (0.1)	10,426 (10.8)	1539 (2.9)	9582 (10.6)	1292 (0.9)	4853 (2.7)
Heart	14 (0.03)	3604 (3.7)	135 (0.3)	2646 (2.9)	40 (0.03)	584 (0.3)
Lung	12 (0.02)	2507 (2.6)	56 (0.1)	2007 (2.2)	1 (0.0)	463 (0.3)
Pancreas	5 (0.01)	1236 (1.3)	24 (0.04)	890 (1.0)	1 (0.0)	143 (0.1)
Small Bowel	0 (0.0)	147 (0.2)	4 (0.01)	43 (0.05)	0 (0.0)	1 (0.0)
Total Organs	**586 (1.2)**	**49,779 (51.4)**	**7885 (14.7)**	**41,299 (45.7)**	**8536 (6.1)**	**18,585 (10.2)**

Table 2.
Absolute numbers and rates of the organ transplant activities per WHO region. 2015 [17].

1.4.2 Dynamics of healthcare

1.4.2.1 Health systems

The WHO defines health systems as "all organizations, people and actions whose primary intent is to promote, restore, or maintain health" [21]. In LRCs, these systems have long been weak and deficient in most aspects of healthcare delivery and therefore, there is persistent need to evaluate health system challenges at all levels [22]. Health security is a crucial public health issue. It is ensured when there is protection against any health threats and also involves ability to handle emerging new health conditions by adapting and developing new approaches [23]. The epidemics in recent years (SARS, MERS and Ebola) including the COVID-19 pandemic bring to the fore the inability of the health systems in SSA to cope with health crisis and other prevalent health conditions [24].

1.4.2.2 Personnel

Some healthcare professionals have poor work ethics deriving from unsavory work environment and remunerations. Transplantation is a highly specialized service that entails full commitment of the workforce and long work hours. For a good transplant programme, the national health system and the hospitals have to commit to improving the skill set of the work force through adequate staff training and other development opportunities, incentivization of the programme and offering a very supportive work environment [25].

1.4.2.3 Health seeking behaviour

Traditions and cultures influence the mindset of a people; decision to access healthcare service is informed by many factors (accessibility, affordability, spirituality and religiosity, and knowledge of the disease condition) [26]. When ill, many people in LRCs seek alternative healthcare service including traditional health providers and religious institutions resulting in late presentation to hospitals [27].

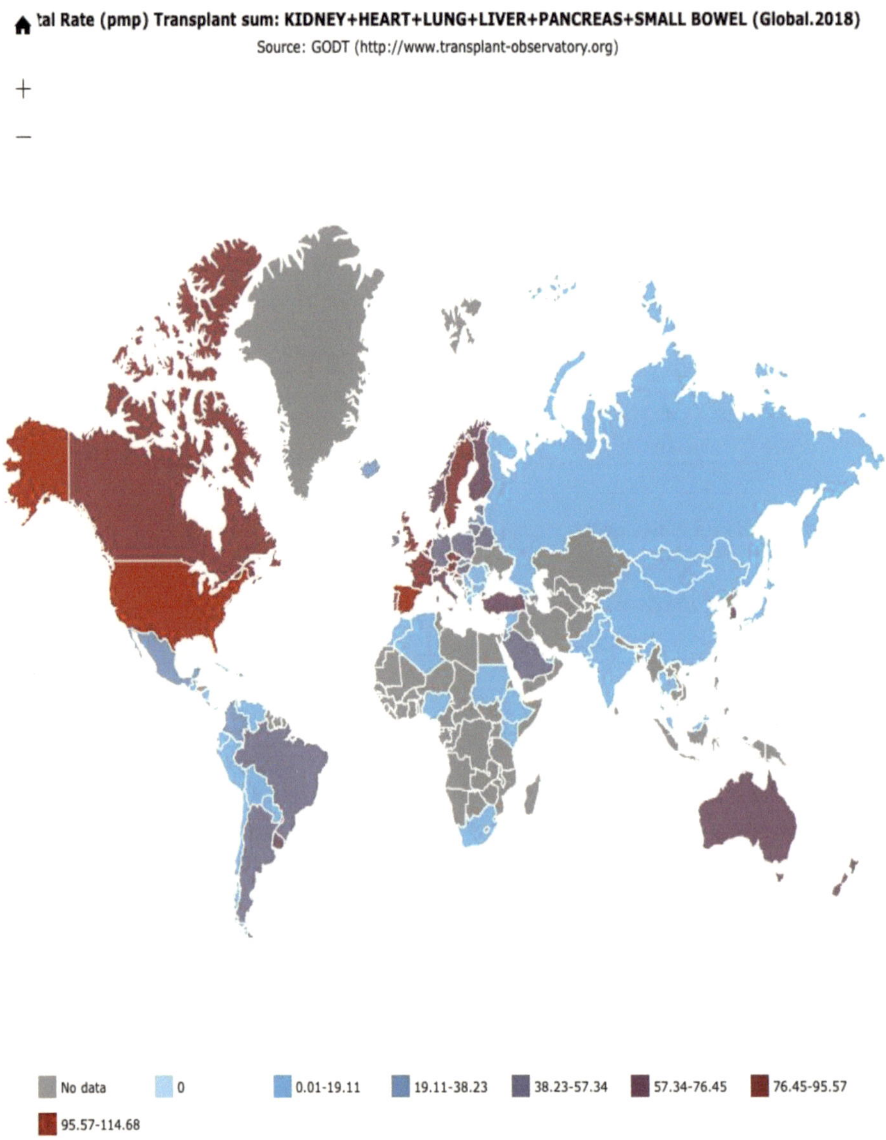

Figure 2.
World map of transplantation in 2019 showing total sum of transplants [from global Observatory of Donation and Transplantation].

1.4.3 Health financing

In 2018 and 2019, Africa's economic growth was at 3.4% and was expected to rise to 3.9% and 4.1% in 2020 and 2021 respectively [28]. Amid the COVID-19 pandemic of 2020, the dynamics changed resulting in contraction of economies globally with expected 1.7% to 3.4% contraction of Africa's economy [29].

The 2001 Abuja Declaration recommended allocation of 15% of the annual national budget to the health sector; achieving this has been challenging [30]. In 2012, 6 countries met the target; and this reduced to 4 in 2014. Currently, the preferred indicator for health financing is the percentage gross domestic product (% GDP). To achieve universal health coverage (UHC), the World Health 2010 Report suggested that a national government has to spend at least 4–5% of GDP on

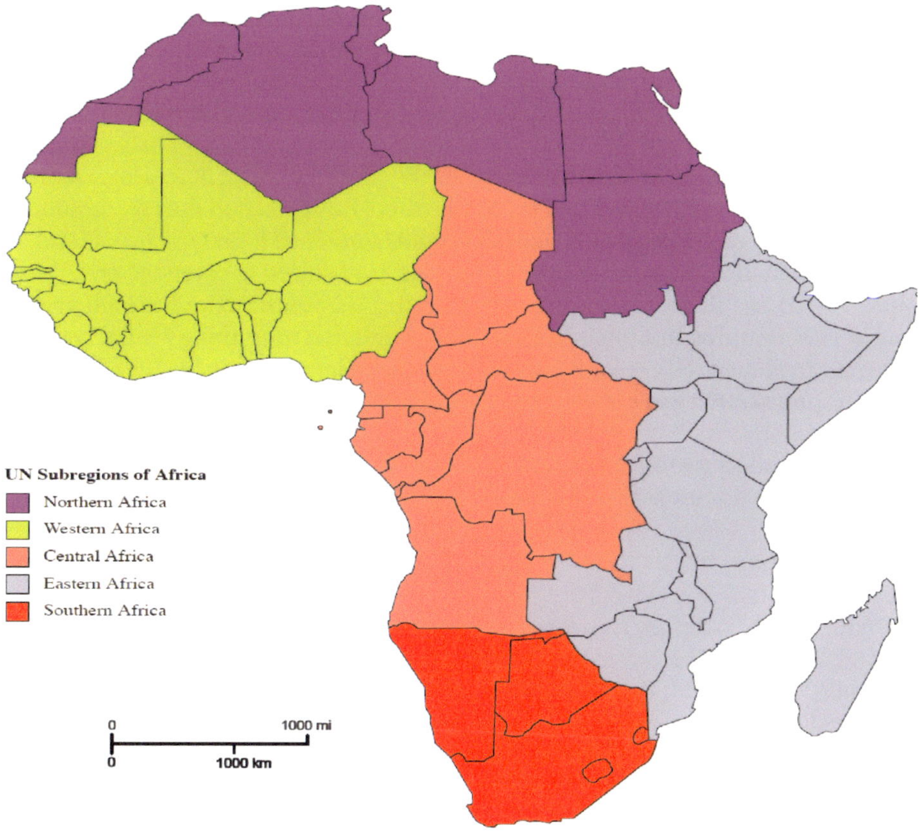

Figure 3.
Map of Africa showing UN sub-regions.

health [31]. Whilst per capita expenditure on health in America and Europe were over $1800 in 2014, the per capita expenditure on health in Africa averaged only $51.6 [32]. Further analysis shows that over the same period, in Africa, general government health expenditure was less than 50% of the total health expenditure while other sources such as out of pocket (OOP) payments and external sources (from funders) accounted for over 50% [32]. In general, transplantation service largely depends on robust and adequate finances hence the programme thrives in HICs and UMICs.

1.5 History of transplantation

1.5.1 Southern Africa

South Africa: the first organ transplantation in Africa was kidney transplant performed by Thomas Starlz and colleagues in 1966 at Wills Donald Gordon Medical Centre, Johannesburg, South Africa [33]. This was followed in 1967 by the first successful heart transplant performed in the world at Groote Shuur Hospital, Cape Town, South Africa by Christian Barnard [34, 35]. Barnard and his team championed the orthotopic and heterotopic ('piggy-back') heart transplant. From 1968 to 1983, they engaged in research on cardiac transplantation thereby laying the foundation for heart transplantation as therapy for end-stage cardiac disease. The team advanced the concept of brain death, organ and tissue donation, and ethical issues in transplantation. They also researched on methods to improve preservation and protection of the donor heart: their studies ranged from developing appropriate hypothermic perfusion for heart storage, haemodynamics and metabolic changes in brain death to xenotransplantation [34].

Though, South Africa has the most advanced transplant programme in the continent, globally, their transplant activities remain lower than those of other countries with comparable economic capacity [35, 36]. South African liver programme has existed for about 2 decades and presently offers living-related liver transplantation. Other solid organ programmes available are combined kidney-pancreas and lung transplantation. Her donor programmes have advanced to extended criteria donors (ECD) and donors after circulatory death [37]. South Africa has high prevalence of HIV resulting in a huge HIV-positive population prompting Muller and colleagues to pioneer HIV-positive-to-positive transplant program in 2008 [38]. By 2018, this programme had successfully transplanted 43 kidneys from 25 deceased donors [39].

Namibia had first kidney transplantation in March 2016 [40] and is also reported to have done a heart transplant [41].

1.5.2 West Africa

Ghana started a kidney transplant programme in 2008 at Korle Bu Teaching Hospital, Accra in collaboration with a hospital and a charity organization in UK. Between 2008 and 2014, the programme performed 17 transplants and in 2015, they established a national registry [42].

Ivory Coast implemented the law authorizing organ donation in 2012 [43] and between 2013 and 2015, ten living-related kidney transplantations had been done [44].

Nigeria commenced organ transplantation activity in 2000 in a privately-owned hospital [45]. Currently, there are 15 centres (public 9, private 6) and over 770 transplants had been performed between 2000 and 2019 [Personal Communication].

1.5.3 East Africa

Ethiopia commenced its transplant programme in collaboration with an American hospital in September 2015 and by February 2018, had done 70 living donor kidney transplants at their only transplant centre [46].

Kenya started kidney transplantation in 2009 and by 2019 had performed 200 transplants. Their government augmented the existing infrastructures to support 10 transplants per month [47].

Mauritius began kidney transplantation in 1980 and discontinued in 1982 following poor outcomes but resumed in 1993 [48]. Although the "Human Tissue (Removal, Preservation and Transplant) Act" was promulgated in 2006 and amended in 2013, a new legislation was enacted in 2018 [49].

Sudan, according to the African Union belongs to East African sub-region even though the United Nations categorized her as North Africa. Sudan had her first kidney transplant in 1974 and for the subsequent 25 years performed very few transplants. However, in 2000, the program was reactivated; and 222 transplants were performed in 2016 [50].

Tanzania started kidney transplantation services locally in collaboration with hospitals in India and Japan in November 2017 [51]. Earlier, her program consisted of government-sponsored transplantation overseas. Recipients and donors received pre-transplantation work-up locally and donor verification by DNA profiling was done to curtail commercialization.

Ugandan cabinet in June 2020 approved a bill to establish a legal framework for human organs, cells and tissue transplant, and to regulate donations and trade in human organs, cells and tissue [52].

1.5.4 Central Africa

No country in this sub-region has a transplant programme but Angola in March 2019 passed a law on human tissue, cell and organ transplant to enable transplantation [53].

In SSA, the national programs for donation and transplantation of organs and tissues are slow and poorly developed and they are fraught with inadequacies in infrastructures, institutional support, and technical expertise [3]. These are attributed to the huge costs and complexity of transplantation, low GDP, lack of subsidy and dearth of facilities.

Loua *et al* in 2018, documented that 62 transplant centres across seven countries in Africa had transplant activities involving kidney, heart, cornea, liver and bone marrow [3].

1.5.5 Stratification of transplant programmes

Programmes are classified into different stages of development of transplant services with those from HICs better developed than those from LMICs and LICs [54] (See **Table 3**).

Stage	Characteristic	Country
I	No existing transplant programme with little or no posttransplant and post-donation care. Transplant tourism is rife.	The poorest countries of the world
II	Faltering or poorly developed transplant programme offering only living-related donation, no nationally structured transplant program, and often no legislation. There is nonexistent deceased-donor program and proliferation of transplant tourism with little or no posttransplant and post-donation care.	Countries in sub-Saharan Africa and many other low- and middle-income countries
III	Fairly developed transplant programme offering mostly living-related donation with rudimentary deceased-donor program. Poorly developed kidney paired exchange and organ sharing programs, often with poor posttransplant and post-donation care. Some level of transplant tourism and moderate to long wait time.	Many countries in Asia, Central and South America, the Middle East, and North Africa
IV	Well-developed structured transplant programme and accompanying legislation offering deceased donation, kidney paired exchange, and organ sharing programs with good posttransplant and post-donation care. Little transplant tourism and short to moderate wait times for transplant.	Many of the developed economies belong to this stage
V	Highly developed and structured transplant programme and accompanying legislation offering mostly deceased donation, advanced donation/kidney paired exchange, and organ sharing programs with excellent posttransplant and post-donation care. There is no transplant tourism and short or no wait times for transplant.	Utopian

Table 3.
Proposed staging for transplant stratification model (transplant transition) [54].

2. Recipient and donor evaluation

2.1 Recipient

Careful evaluation of potential organ transplant recipients is necessary to detect co-existing illnesses that can adversely affect the prognosis of the transplantation. The subsisting clinical practice guidelines including the 2020 KDIGO guideline and the 2011 UK Renal Association Clinical Practice guideline (5th Edition) [55, 56] recommend the standard process of evaluation of prospective transplant recipients. Regardless of the recommendations of the practice guidelines, most transplant centres have their in-house protocols for transplant recipient evaluation. However, in SSA, the evaluation may be tailored to the available resources but should be efficient and cost-effective. The discussion below is typical for kidney transplant units in Nigeria but may apply to other organ transplantations and transplantations in other countries in the sub-region.

The evaluation of such candidates involves risk/benefit assessment and they should have at least five-year life expectancy derived from age, gender and race of the individual [57]. Many clinicians, however, consider other factors including severity of life-threatening diseases, functional status, clinical experience and knowledge of the patient to determine suitability for organ transplantation.

2.1.1 Workup for transplant candidates

The workup evaluation includes: hematological, clinical chemistry, infection profile, diagnostic procedures, imaging and immunological tests. The list of relevant investigations is shown in **Table 4**.

2.1.1.1 Hematological studies

Blood grouping establishes the candidate's blood type and determines if further evaluation should proceed. Recipient and donor must be compatible. Complete blood count and clotting profile should be optimal.

2.1.1.2 Cardiac evaluation

All candidates are assessed for presence of cardiac disease by history, physical examination and electrocardiogram. Recipients with cardiac disease, comorbidities that predispose to coronary artery disease (CAD), history of previous CAD or poor cardiac function are further assessed by cardiologists. Generally, contraindications for transplantation include severe heart disease (New York Heart Association [NYHA] Functional Class III/IV), severe CAD, left ventricular dysfunction [ejection fraction <30%] and severe valvular disease.

2.1.1.3 Pulmonary evaluation

Chest radiograph is required for all candidates while chest computerized tomography (CT) is reserved for current or former heavy smokers ($\geq$ 30 pack-years). Candidates with lung disease are further evaluated by a pulmonologist. Severe irreversible obstructive or restrictive pulmonary diseases are contraindications for transplantation.

Blood	1. Complete blood count and differential 2. Blood group 3. INR, PTT 4. Tissue typing: CDC and flow cytometry 5. Electrolytes: sodium, potassium, calcium, magnesium 6. Kidney function: urea, creatinine 7. Liver function: bilirubin, total protein, albumin, alkaline phosphatase, ALT, AST, LDH, GGT 8. Fasting blood glucose, glycated hemoglobin 9. Total cholesterol, HDL, LDL, VLDL, TG 10. Serology: HIV, HBsAg, Anti HCV, CMV, syphilis, EBV, HSV
Radiology	1. Chest radiograph 2. Abdominal and pelvic ultrasound. 3. CT angiography
Urine	1. Urinalysis 2. Urine MCS
Immunology	1. HLA typing, HLA antibodies, crossmatching
Gynecological	1. Pap smear, mammogram for women >40 years or family history of breast cancer
Other tests	1. Electrocardiogram 2. Echocardiography 3. Colonoscopy if >50 years 4. PSA in men >50 years

Table 4.
Workup for prospective organ transplant recipients.

2.1.1.4 Tuberculosis screening

Sub-Saharan Africa has high prevalence of tuberculosis (TB). It is therefore necessary to screen for TB in prospective organ recipients with a chest radiograph and purified protein derivative (PPD) skin test. Candidates with positive TB screening tests are treated before organ transplantation.

2.1.1.5 Gastrointestinal evaluation

Candidates with history of peptic ulcer disease (PUD) are screened with oesophagogastroscopy and *Helicobacter pylori* test. Active diseases including PUD, diverticulitis, pancreatitis, cholelithiasis and inflammatory bowel disease should be controlled before transplantation.

2.1.1.6 Serologies

Serological tests for potentially transmissible diseases, like HIV, HBV, HCV, cytomegalovirus (CMV), Epstein–Barr virus and varicella-zoster virus are usually performed, and appropriate management instituted when indicated.

2.1.1.7 Cancer screening

Routine cancer screening is done for all recipients. Chest radiograph is mandatory while chest CT is reserved for current or former heavy smokers. Ultrasonography is used for screening candidates at risk of renal cell carcinoma (dialysis >3 years, family history of renal cancer, acquired cystic disease, analgesic nephropathy). Those at risk of urinary bladder cancer (high-level exposure to cyclophosphamide, heavy smoking) require cystoscopy. Patients at risk of hepato-cellular carcinoma are screened with ultrasonography and serum alpha fetoprotein. Colonoscopy is done to screen for bowel cancer and inflammatory bowel disease. Females undergo PAP smear and mammography to exclude cervical and breast cancer respectively.

2.1.2 Obesity

Obesity increases the risk of post-operative complications. Many transplant centres prefer a body mass index (BMI) of <30.

2.1.3 Financial considerations and psychosocial status

These are very important aspects of the workup for prospective organ transplant recipients and will be discussed later.

2.2 Donor

Donor protection should always be taken into account during living donor selection and assessment. Organ donation should be altruistic, voluntary and never coerced. Donor evaluation is a multidisciplinary exercise, and is done before, during and after donation. Due to lack of requisite legislation, supporting infra-structure, religious and cultural beliefs, mostly living organ donations are done in SSA countries.

There are risks associated with organ donation and consequently, potential donors should receive medical, surgical and psychological screening. Pre, intra, and post-operative care as well as structured post-donation follow up are important.

2.2.1 Clinical evaluation

Potential donors should be healthy and neither too young nor too old. Medical history and physical examination could elicit risk factors for kidney disease such as: DM, hypertension, family history of kidney disease, herbal drug, non-steriodal anti-inflammatory drugs (NSAIDs), and other nephrotoxin use. History and/or presence of CLD could be suggested by jaundice and alcohol abuse. Also, history of psychiatric illness, malignancies, smoking and substance abuse, etc. should be sought and positive candidates excluded. Donors should not be morbidly obese and blood pressures should be <140/90 mmHg.

2.2.1.1 Donor work-up

For various investigations see **Table 5**.

Absence of urinary markers of disease such as proteinuria, haematuria, pyuria and casts, may rule out kidney diseases in potential donors. Glomerular filtration rate (GFR) should ideally be measured but is often estimated using serum cre-atinine in most LRCs. Prospective donors are screened for chronic viral diseases.

Parameters	Relevant indices
Age	>18, <60 years
History	Diabetes mellitus, hypertension, nephrotoxins, alcohol and other substance abuse, cigarette smoking, psychiatric illness, malignancy
Physical features	Jaundice, pallor, BP >140/90 mmHg, BMI >35
Laboratory features	
Hematological	FBC, PT/INR
Chemistry	SEUCr, LFT, lipid profile, FBG, HBA1C, PSA, TFT
Microbiology	Urinalysis, urine culture
Serological/ immunological	HIV, Anti HCV, HBsAg, CMV, EBV, ABO blood group, HLA A, B and DR matching, HLA antibody cross- matching
Imaging	Ultrasound, CT angiography,
Others	ECG, Echocardiography

Table 5.
Workup for potential organ transplant donors.

Notably, CMV positivity in a donor has implication for a CMV-negative recipient, who due to subsequent immunosuppressive drug use will likely succumb to its infection. Screening for TB (CXR, Mantoux test, sputum GeneXpert) is important in SSA because 1/3 of the population is infected with M. tuberculosis [58]. The ABO blood group compatibility with recipient is mandatory; however, Rhesus factor mismatch is not a major consideration for solid organ matching. There are many HLA antigens (Class I: HLA-A, B, and C; Class II: HLA-DR, DQ and DP), but the HLA A, B and DR are usually cross-matched between donors and recipients (i.e. tissue typing).HLA antibody cross-matching is important to prevent early graft rejection. It detects the presence of HLA antibodies in recipients that can react with donor's lymphocytes, i.e. donor specific antibodies (DSA).

HLA antibody cross-matching was originally based on complement dependent cytotoxicity (CDC) assays. It is done with recipient's serum on donor lymphocytes or pooled lymphocytes of previous donors within the transplant centre's population to determine the Panel Reactive Antibodies (PRA). Reactive Antibodies (PRA). The PRA estimates the recipient's chances of tolerating allografts from that population and is useful for deceased donation.

Solid phase assays, ELISA or flow cytometry (Luminex)-based are now available and preferred. Most transplant centres in SSA, outsource tissue typing and HLA antibody cross-matching. Protocols require at least two HLA antibody cross-matches, with the last, just before the transplant procedure.

Imaging evaluation using ultrasonography and doppler in prospective donors should demonstrate normal kidneys (sizes and echotexture) and renal blood flow.

The CT-angiography helps to rule out solitary kidney or detect the presence of multiple or abnormal renal arteries, which have surgical implications for nephrectomy in donors and anastomoses in recipients.

2.2.2 Counseling

Counseling donors on short and long-term risks associated with organ donation is necessary. Possible complications such as pain, post-operative infections, blood loss, deep venous thrombosis and pulmonary embolism can occur. Studies have shown that peri-operative mortality and morbidity during organ donation, are about 0.03% and 10% respectively [59]. Some studies show that with careful selection, kidney donors live long, although hypertension, proteinuria and reduced GFR can occur over time [60]. The risk of ESKD following kidney donation is about 0.3% [61]. Emotional consequences after organ donation should be anticipated therefore psychosocial assessment should be independently organized by the transplant team before and after donation.

2.3 Post donation follow-up

Many transplantation programmes in SSA adopt protocols from established and experienced centres.

According to US Organ Procurement and Transplantation Network (OPTN) guidelines, living donor follow-up is done at discharge (or at 6 weeks), 1 year and 2 years [62]. Parameters monitored include weight, blood pressure, lipid profile, kidney and liver functions. Healthy eating, regular exercise and the dangers of substance abuse are emphasized. After uneventful 2 years, donor follow-up is continued by the primary care physicians but for those with adverse outcomes appropriate referral is made. Post-donation follow-up is important for donor safety and wellbeing to enable diagnosis and treatment of co-morbidities.

2.4 Psychosocial evaluation

In transplantation, recipients, donors and their families are faced with various challenges including psychological and behavioral issues. Evaluation is essential in the following aspects: candidate and donor selection, counseling, pre- and post-transplant assessment, patient, caregiver and family adjustments to transplant and issues related to psyche of transplant staff.

2.4.1 Recipient

Various factors exert neuropsychiatric effects in transplantation. Studies link significant neuropsychiatric adverse effects to cyclosporine, tacrolimus, steroids and other components of treatment. Therefore, psychosocial issues should be considered and addressed in order to achieve a successful transplant.

Psychosocial evaluation of patients for transplant include [63]:

- Patient profile: relationships, education, work and legal history
- Expectations from the surgery
- Organ failure: cause, complications, course, adherence to treatment
- Ways of coping with the illness
- Support network: caregivers, family, friends, faith organizations and employers
- Psychiatric history: extant, past and family.
- Substance abuse history
- Mental status exam: neuropsychiatric tests
- Ability to give informed consent

There are known stressors before and after transplantation including depression and hopelessness, anxiety, uncertainty and aggression. These may be followed by hope, and confidence in an unpredictable pattern as recipients gradually process adaptation to the new situation.

After Transplantation, recipients pass through three phases of adaptation [64]:

- "Foreign body" phase: the organ feels strange to the recipient. Persecution anxiety or idealization could arise. The organ could be seen as fragile and precious, thereby generating excessive protective feelings towards it.
- "Partial incorporation" phase: recipient begins to integrate the organ.
- "Total incorporation" phase: recipient is no longer aware of the organ.

In the long-term postoperative period, medication side effects and associated comorbidities become central stressors affecting the recipients' quality of life (QOL). The most bothersome stressors are work related, like farming, schooling, etc. [65]. Recipients might feel stressed by the strict adherence to the medical regimen. This, in turn, can compromise their adherence after transplantation. Financial problems and legal disputes constitute other possible sources of psychological strain with health or pension insurance agencies, where available.

Enabling transplant recipients commence productive employment constitutes the main goal of transplantation and is considered an indicator of societal participation [66]. Globally, data show that 18% - 86% of recipients return to work or find new employment. [67, 68] but no data is available for SSA.

2.4.2 Donor

2.4.2.1 Donors' motives and decision-making

Multiple factors motivating donors include intrinsic factors (e.g., desire to relieve another's suffering or to act in accordance with religious convictions) and extrinsic factors (social pressures or perceived norms) that may operate simultaneously. The combination of motivational forces differs depending on whether and how the donor is related to the recipient.

Most living donors use two decision-making strategies: [69]: "moral" which involves awareness that one's actions can affect another [70] and "rational" which is focused on gathering relevant information, evaluating alternatives, selecting an alternative, and implementing the decision.

2.4.2.2 Psychological status and post-donation psychosocial outcomes

Potential donors' psychological stability has been one of the greatest concerns for living transplant programmes, particularly in the context of unrelated donation. The willingness or desire to donate to a stranger has been historically viewed with suspicion [71, 72]. Studies suggest that most potential donors do not suffer from mental illness [73, 74]. Many donors have reported positive feelings about donation however, a few have observed psychological distress, anxiety and depression. Thus, it becomes critical to identify, and mitigate key risk factors for these poorer outcomes: non-first degree relatives [75, 76], ambivalent donors [76, 77] and "black sheep" donors (persons who donate in order to compensate for past wrong doings or to restore their position in the family) are at higher risk for poorer post-donation psychosocial outcomes [76, 77].

3. Surgical aspect of transplantation

3.1 Donor surgery

The donor kidney angiogram is decisive in selecting the kidney to be harvested. The larger kidney with better blood flow is left for the donor. Minimal access donor nephrectomy and robot-assisted renal engraftment reduce postoperative complications. These, however, are not easily available in most LRCs.

3.1.1 Complications of donor nephrectomy

Post-operative donor complications occur in 7.9–22% with bleeding in about 3%. Infectious, gastrointestinal, respiratory, cardiac and psychiatric complications may occur [78–80].

3.2 Recipient surgery

The harvested kidney is covered in ice slush, wrapped in gauze piece and preserved in ice container as organ perfusion machine is not readily available in the sub-region.

Kidneys with multiple arteries are avoided but if inevitable, arteries are anastomosed side to side, end to side, or separately onto the external iliac artery (**Figure 4**). The right external iliac vessels are more superficial than the left and this side is frequently preferred for the first renal engraftment.

Anti-reflux uretero-cystostomy is performed over a size 4Fg double J-ureteric stent (**Figure 5**).

3.2.1 Pitfall in recipients surgery

Sclerosed External Iliac Vein (EIV): this results from repeated cannulation of EIV for hemodialysis. Recipient pre-operative EIV doppler ultrasound scan for patency is important. Major complications of recipient engraftment include bleeding, delayed graft function, hyperacute rejection and allograft renal vein thrombosis.

3.3 Peri and post-operative care of renal transplant recipient

Immunosuppressive regimen is divided into induction and maintenance phases.

3.3.1 Induction phase

This is required to prevent acute rejection. Due to sensitization from blood transfusions, previous pregnancies (females) and increased susceptibility to graft rejection (in blacks) recipients undergo induction [81]. A combination of antithymocyte globulin (ATG) and methylprednisolone is often used. Prior to this, patients receive pretreatment with acetaminophen and antihistamines to prevent cytokine release syndrome associated with ATG.

Biologic agents (Alemtuzumab, Basiliximab, Daclizumab) may be used when available in less sensitized patients.

3.3.2 Maintenance regimen

To prevent allograft rejection, maintenance immunosuppression is achieved with a combination of low dose corticosteroid (prednisolone is widely in available SSA), an antiproliferative agent (mycophenolate mofetil (MMF) or azathioprine)

DOI: http://dx.doi.org/10.5772/intechopen.94986

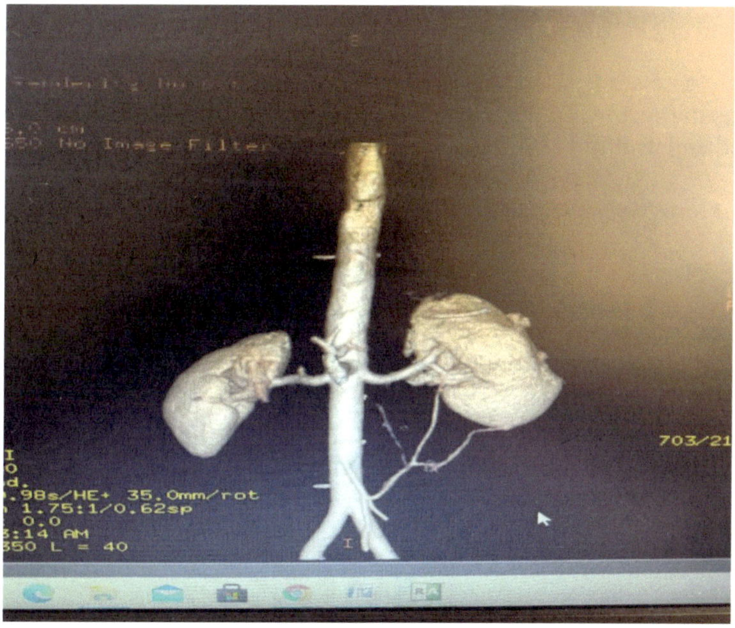

Figure 4.
Donor angiogram with multiple left renal arteries.

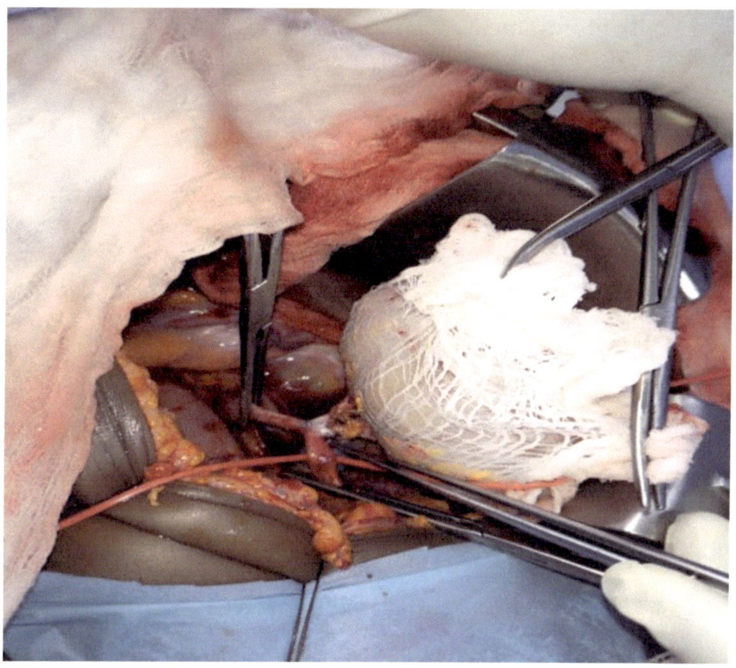

Figure 5.
End-to-side donor-recipient arterial anastomosis with kidney wrapped in gauze piece packed with saline ice slush.

and a calcineurin inhibitor (CNI) (tacrolimus (TAC) or cyclosporine (CYP)). Tacrolimus has shown superiority over cyclosporine in improving graft survival and preventing acute rejection. Thus, TAC remains an integral part of the common post-transplant immunosuppressive combination [82]. The initiating dose is titrated to achieve a trough level of 8-10 ng/ml in the first three months post-transplant.

Prophylaxis against bacteria, fungi and viruses are commenced within this time.

3.3.2.1 First post-operative week

First day post-surgery, emphasis is on haemodynamic and respiratory stability as well as urine output. By the first week, good graft function should have been established and urethral catheter is removed.

3.3.2.2 First three post-operative months

Within this period opportunistic infections are anticipated and appropriate measures taken. The ureteric stent is removed within 4 – 6 weeks.

3.4 Transplant outcomes in SSA

Absence of transplant registries in SSA precludes transplant data availability. However, between 2010 and 2015, a hospital in South Africa documented recipient survival at 1 and 5 years as 90.4% and 83.1% and that of graft 89.4% and 80% respectively [83].

4. Challenges of transplantation

Organ donation and transplantation in SSA is fraught with numerous challenges including costs of treatment, inadequate infrastructure and equipment, dearth of highly skilled health professionals, and lack of well-articulated ethico-legal framework and policies [3].

4.1 Cost of treatment

Cost of kidney transplant varies from country to country. For example, the cost is estimated at about $32,000 in Nigeria [84], $18,775 in Ghana [85], and $10,000 in Tanzania [20].

Source of funding for organ and tissue donation and transplant depends on the country: public sources in Ethiopia, Ghana, Mali, Seychelles and Comoros but private in Nigeria, Burkina Faso, Madagascar and 10 other countries See **Table 6**. Most recipients pay OOP either personally or by relatives, employers and to a lesser extent philanthropists [45]. While the National insurance pays two-thirds of the transplant cost in Kenya [47], it is free in Tanzania [51].

Post-transplant maintenance of immunosuppression is a major challenge. This is exigent since therapy must be individualized. Two perspectives associated with immunosuppression in SSA include:

- Availability, affordability and patient's adherence to prescription.

- Therapeutic drug monitoring (TDM).

4.1.1 Availability, affordability and patient's adherence to prescription

Adequate immunosuppression is key to allograft survival. In patients who pay OOP, prohibitive costs of medications may have negative impact on their finances. Furthermore, side effects of medications affect their health-related QOL. In many LRCs, these medicines are imported at high cost and not readily available. These contribute to poor adherence with subsequent allograft rejection and graft loss.

Indicator	Countries
Countries with functional transplantation programmes	
Functional transplantation programmes from living donors	Algeria, Côte d'Ivoire, Ethiopia, Ghana, Kenya, Namibia, Nigeria, United Republic of Tanzania, Uganda, South Africa
No. of transplant centres in the region	
Kidney centres	Algeria, Côte d'Ivoire, Ethiopia, Ghana, Kenya, Namibia, Nigeria, United Republic of Tanzania, Uganda
Corneal centres	Kenya, Nigeria, South Africa
Bone marrow centres	Nigeria, South Africa
Liver centres	South Africa
Heart centres	South Africa, others perform open heart surgeries
Countries having legal requirements	
Legal requirements in place covering organ donations and/or transplantations	Burkina Faso, Comoros, Côte d'Ivoire, Ethiopia, Kenya, Mauritius, Namibia, Nigeria, Rwanda, Senegal, Sudan, United Republic of Tanzania, Uganda, Zimbabwe
Governments intended to adopt new legal requirements	Cameroon, Chad, Eswatini, Ghana, Guinea, Madagascar, Mali, Mozambique
No legislations in place	Angola, Benin, Burundi, Cabo Verde, Congo, Eritrea, Gabon, Guinea Bissau, Seychelles, Sierra Leone
Legal requirements in place to inform living donors on the risks of the operation	Comoros, Ethiopia, Kenya, Mali, Nigeria, Rwanda, Senegal, Seychelles, United Republic of Tanzania, Uganda
Legal restrictions on the coverage of donation costs for living donors	Comoros, Mali, Rwanda, Senegal
Legal requirement to follow-up on the outcomes of living donors	Ethiopia, Mali, Senegal, Seychelles
Legal requirement to provide care to living donors in case of adverse or medical consequences	Ethiopia, Senegal, Seychelles
Prohibition of organ trafficking/transplant commercialization	Burkina Faso, Comoros, Côte d'Ivoire, Mali, Namibia, Nigeria, Rwanda, Senegal
Legal permit and regulation of financial incentives for living donors	None
Import or export of organs authorized	Ghana, Namibia, Rwanda
Import or export of organs explicitly prohibited	Burkina Faso, Seychelles
Legal requirements for organ and tissue donations from living donors[a]	Burkina Faso, Comoros, Côte d'Ivoire, Kenya, Mali, Nigeria, Rwanda, Senegal, Seychelles, United Republic of Tanzania, Uganda
No. of countries having an organization and management system	
Authorization for transplant services	Burkina Faso, Comoros, Côte d'Ivoire, Ethiopia, Ghana, Guinea, Kenya, Madagascar, Mali, Nigeria, Senegal, Uganda, Zimbabwe
Ethics Committees at the national or local level	Burkina Faso, Comoros, Côte d'Ivoire, Ethiopia, Gabon, Kenya, Mali, Nigeria, Rwanda, Senegal
Government recognized authority at the national level	Algeria, Côte d'Ivoire, Ethiopia, Ghana, Kenya, Mali, Nigeria, Senegal, Uganda
Setting up protocols, guidelines, recommendations	Comoros, Côte d'Ivoire, Ethiopia, Mali, Senegal

Indicator	Countries
Transplant follow-up registries for post-transplant living donor and for recipients	Côte d'Ivoire, Ethiopia, Namibia, Uganda
Affiliation with an international organ allocation organization	None
Cooperation framework to allow transplantation abroad	Côte d'Ivoire, Ethiopia, Kenya, Namibia, United Republic of Tanzania, Uganda
Training programme for staff in place	Côte d'Ivoire, Ethiopia
Source of funding	
Public	Comoros, Ethiopia, Ghana, Mali, Seychelles, United Republic of Tanzania
Private	Côte d'Ivoire, Ghana, Nigeria
Public and Private	Kenya, Namibia, South Africa, Uganda
Not Specified	Eswatini, Gabon, Zimbabwe

Table 6.
Aspects of transplantation programmes in SSA modified from Loua et al [3].

4.2 Therapeutic drug monitoring (TDM)

Despite their impactful role in improving transplant outcome and graft survival, immunosuppressive medicines exhibit narrow therapeutic range between levels that inhibit rejection and toxic levels hence TDM is often required. Establishing a patient's dose requirements in the immediate post – surgery period and avoiding over immunosuppression remains a challenge. Calcineurin inhibitors have variable pharmacokinetics [86–89]. While ethnic differences have not been demonstrated in pharmacokinetics of MMF and AZA, African Americans have been shown to have 20–50% lower oral bioavailability for TAC, CYP, sirolimus and everolimus and as such require higher drug doses than Caucasians [90, 91]. This has been attributed to genetic polymorphism of key enzymes in the metabolism of these medications [90]. Genetic profiling is not readily done in SSA hence, TDM is essential. This attracts huge costs for the health system and for patients who pay OOP. It is imperative to tailor medications to patient's need. Some countries do not have the capacity to analyze drug levels, so patient's blood samples are sent overseas for analysis. Within the first-year post-transplant, TDM is done at least twice during timed follow-up visit for patients coming from rural and urban areas. However, more frequent monitoring is done when indicated. During emergency presentation for allograft dysfunction, patients are admitted, samples for TDM sent out and other possible causes of allograft dysfunction are excluded or managed if present. Decision to increase drug dosage is often delayed till TDM result is available but dose reduction or withdrawal can be done in the presence of overt signs and symptoms suggestive of toxicity. For subsequent years, TDM is done as indicated.

4.3 Lack of infrastructure and equipment

Tissue typing, cross-matching and some viral studies, which are major aspects of patient preparation, are done overseas. This tends to delay the procedure and leads to an increase in the cost of transplantation. Adequate histological evaluation of biopsy specimens are largely unavailable, making prompt management of rejections and infections problematic.

4.4 Dearth of skilled transplant workforce

Health-workforce is the backbone of any health care system. Transplantation involves collaboration of many health professionals (nephrologists, transplant surgeons, urologists, renal nurses, pathologists, etc.). Worldwide transplant workforce and training capacity remain unknown. Of the 47 countries in SSA, only 15 (32.6%) had data on the number of nephrologists in their countries. Nigeria and South Africa have the greatest number of nephrologists with rates <10 per 10,000 population while others have < two per 10,000 population [3]. The situation is worse for other specialists involved in transplantation. Opportunities for training and employment have caused brain drain to developed countries from LRCs [3].

4.5 Transplant programmes

Despite the burden of ESKD in SSA, only few countries have sustained transplant programmes [20]. There are only 62 centres across 7 countries in SSA [3]. Nigeria with a population of 206 million has 15 renal transplant centres (RTCs) with majority recording low activities ranging 1–5 transplants per year (Personal Communication). South Africa with a population of 59.37 million (2020) has 14 RTCs and did 250 to 450 kidney transplants annually between 1991 and 2015 [35].

4.6 Shortage of organs

Scarcity of organs for transplantation is a multi-factorial global problem. Living donors remain the major source of organs for transplantation in SSA with largely non-existent deceased donor programmes. This has resulted in the persistent dearth of organs in the face of continuous rise in demand [92]. Unavailable storage facilities, poor knowledge about transplantation, socio-cultural and religious beliefs (which discourage living organ donation, view deceased organ donation as a taboo or an act of mutilating the dead with violation of the person's dignity [84]) contribute to shortage of organs [93].

4.7 Poverty and unemployment

There is pervading poverty in SSA with US bureau of statistics reporting rates of 87.8%, 56.9%, 40.1%, 40% and 36.1% in Uganda, Ghana, Nigeria, Cameroun and Kenya respectively [94]. In Nigeria, 85% of ESKD patients earn between $800–7333 annually making kidney transplantation unaffordable [27, 95]. Although unemployment rate in SSA averages 6.2%, many are underemployed and earn low income [96].

4.8 Poor accessibility

Most transplant centres are located in urban cities or state capitals reducing accessibility to rural dwellers [3, 41].

4.9 Cultural and religious considerations

Christianity, Islam and African traditional religion are the major faiths in SSA. Interplay of faith, religion and cultural attitudes and their relationship with views on organ donation is complex. Response to illness as God's will negates organ donation or reception. Belief in resurrection and reincarnation precludes organ donation since the 'new body' may have some missing parts. Desecration of the body of the deceased is reported as a factor prohibiting family members from donating body parts of their deceased relatives.

4.10 Poor coordination and management

Functional organizational mechanism for transplant programmes including authorization for transplant services; ethics committees, guidelines and protocols, etc. are few in the region [41, 93]. Additionally, transplant is not sufficiently integrated into national health services and collaboration between SSA countries is limited.

Absence of functional and reliable registries militate against planning and implementation of policies due to lack of data. Most countries do not include performance indicators for organ donation and transplantation in their national health information systems. In addition, there is insufficient multisectoral (schools, transport departments, NGOs, Civil Society Organizations, etc.) involvement in transplantation programmes in SSA.

4.11 Legal and regulatory policies

Some countries have legislation for organ donation and transplantation while others are in various stages of developing theirs (**Table 6**). The weak regulatory frameworks observed in these countries are often insufficient to ensure the effective oversight needed for the implementation of quality standards for organ transplantation.

4.12 Transplant tourism (TT)

The Declaration of Istanbul defines organ transplant tourism as travel for transplantation involving trafficking in persons, for the purpose of organ removal. Organ trafficking is defined as *"the recruitment, transport, transfer, harboring, or receipt of living or deceased persons or their organs by means of any form of coercion, of abduction, of fraud, of deception, of the abuse of power or of a position of vulnerability, or of the giving to, or the receiving by, a third party of payments, or benefits to achieve the transfer of control over the potential donor for the purpose of exploitation by the removal of organs for transplantation* [97]." Transplant commercialism is the buying and selling of organs i.e. treating of organs as commodities. Travel for transplantation is the transport of organs, donors, recipients, or the professionals across borders for transplantation and it becomes TT if it entails organ trafficking and/or transplant commercialism [97]. Transplant tourism has become an increasing component of medical tourism (MT) especially in SSA. The disparity between the demand for and supply of organs encourages illegal organ procurement as transplantation may the only life-saving treatment in many end-organ failure. Unavailability and high cost of healthcare, lack of faith in local health systems, widening economic gap, ease of global travel and uneven global application of laws, have led to increase in TT.

5. Transplant opportunities

Transplantation holds lots of opportunities which if well harnessed can improve healthcare in SSA.

5.1 Availability of organs for transplantation

For sustainable transplantation programme, individuals, community and governmental commitment and collaboration are required. Availability of organs can be increased through heightened public enlightenment campaigns emphasizing preventive medicine and change in the community's organ donation perception. This can be achieved by partnering with religious bodies, individual, family and community education, inclusion of transplantation and donation in school syllabus, alliance with the department of motor vehicles (DMV) and novel donation programmes (kidney paired donation, extended criteria organ donation and altruistic non-directed donation).

5.2 Comprehensive legislation and regulation

Transplantation has significant medico-legal implications requiring robust legal framework. This should cover organ donation legitimacy, regulatory bodies, criteria and processes of accreditation, certification and standardization of transplant centres [98]. Transplantation programmes afford SSA opportunities to learn and adapt legislation from other regions. In 2008, Israeli parliament accepted two laws from their Ministry of Health - the Brain-Respiratory Death for determination of brain death and the Organ transplantation laws [99]. These laws defined the ethical, legal and organizational aspects of organ donation, allocation and transplantation with prioritization of registered donors, donor reimbursement and life insurance [99]. These and stoppage of illegal TT reimbursement significantly increased living and deceased organ donation by 2011 [99, 100].

5.3 Manpower development

The Multidisciplinary nature of transplant programmes demands highly skilled manpower often not obtainable in many parts of SSA, hence the need for collaboration with advanced transplant centres. Such patnership enables capacity development and training of specialized workforce which will serve the local and sister institutions.

5.4 Transplant protocols and registry

Successful transplantation requires protocols for recipient and donor care. Transplant centres in LRCs can develop or adapt protocols from advanced centres, international organizations like United Network for Organ Sharing, Donation and Transplant Institute etc. National registries of organ transplant and outcomes are essential for documentation of transplant activities, reporting of short and long-term outcomes, and for planning and budgeting.

5.5 Developing transplant programmes

Each country should establish a sustainable transplant programme. Development of such services will curb organ trafficking and TT [101]. It entails infrastructural, legislative and manpower development with national government's political will [35, 102]. A well-defined mode of funding which includes transplantation in national health insurance coverage ensures sustainability.

Transplantation programme can be established in a staged fashion [101]: enacting transplantation related laws and regulations, capacity building, extensive public enlightenment campaigns and transplant beginning with live-donor and subsequently, deceased-donor.

5.5.1 Transplant models

Models that can be adapted include:

5.5.1.1 The Pakistani model

In the Pakistani model [103, 104], following intense public enlightenment, the community assumed ownership of the programme through donations as individuals, communities and NGOs. Government provided 30–40% of required cost, infrastructure, staff training and emolument enabling patients to receive free nephrology and transplantation care plus post-transplant rehabilitation. Accountability, transparency and equity ensured the success of this model.

5.5.1.2 Iranian model

Following development of indigenous transplant programme in 1985, there was an unwieldy transplant waiting list necessitating government-sponsored live-unrelated transplant with donor compensation [105]. This programme successfully eliminated waiting list by 1999 increasing kidney transplantation to 28 pmp per year. The Dialysis and Transplant Patients Association facilitated donor-recipient matching excluding third party. Donors also received government-funded life health insurance and gifts. Government additionally supported importation and free distribution of immunosuppressive medications to recipients. Deceased donor transplantation has steadily increased since 2000.

These models emphasize the indispensable roles of community, government and NGOs in ensuring the existence of a sustainable transplantation programme.

6. Other aspects of transplantation in sub-Saharan Africa: guidance efforts by international organization

The World Health Assembly (WHA) adopted resolutions WHA57.18 and WHA63.22 [106, 107], and the WHO guiding principles on human cell, tissue and organ transplantation to guide transplantation programmes and activities [108]. The United Nations General assembly adopted these resolutions to strengthen and promote effective measures and international cooperation to prevent and combat organ trafficking [109]. The Istanbul declaration on organ trafficking and TT recommends a legal and professional framework to govern organ donation and transplantation activities, transparent regulatory oversight system to ensure donor and recipient safety, enforce standards and prohibit unethical practices in all countries [97]. A Task Force to check unwholesome practices in transplantation was set up and inaugurated by WHO in 2017 [110].

During the 2013 Global Alliance of Transplantation (GAT) meeting organized by Southern African Transplant Society in Durban [3], the transplantation society (TTS) sponsored a meeting for countries in SSA to assess the need for and ability to optimize or develop local transplant programmes. In 2015, the South African Renal Society–African Association of Nephrology in collaboration with European Renal Association-European Dialysis and Transplant Association held a pre-congress workshop to encourage SSA countries to develop renal registries [111]. Attempts at establishing renal registries in SSA have met with challenges. The International Society of Nephrology (ISN) is supporting establishment of renal registries worldwide through her SHARing Expertise (https://www.theisn.org/initiatives/data-collection/). Leveraging on such programmes can help SSA countries establish reliable registries.

To improve kidney disease patients' care and capacity building worldwide, ISN pioneers these programs: fellowship, ISN continuing medical education, sister renal centre (SRC), sister transplant centre (STC) and educational ambassadors programme. Through ISN- TTS-STC program, ISN encourages establishment and development of transplant centres (www.theisn.org/programs). In ISN- TTS STC programme, SSA centres (emerging centres) can partner with developed centres (supporting centre) for capacity building through institutional and exchange training programmes at no cost to the individual or his home institution. This partnership is superior to the intermittent use of paid expatriates in some SSA countries.

7. Recommendations

Improvement in the transplant landscape of SSA can be achieved by adapting models that have proven successful in LRCs such as those of Pakistan and Iran. Implementing the 2007 World Health Organization Regional Consultation recommendations: establishment of national legal framework and self-sufficient organ donation and transplantation in each country, transparent transplantation practices, and prevention of commercialized transplantation and TT will improve transplantation programmes in SSA. Also, adopting the WHO Regional Committee for Africa's proposed actions on organ transplantation for member states and establishment of national registries for organ transplantation in each country are needed.

8. Conclusion

Sub-Saharan Africa, comprising of 47 countries and occupying an area of about 24 million Km^2 is heterogeneous with estimated population of 1.1 billion people. Most of the countries belong to the LICs and LMICs according to World Bank Classification of economies. This region has a high prevalence of end-organ diseases including CKD, CLD, chronic lung diseases and chronic heart diseases resulting from CDs and NCDs.

Although South Africa performed Africa's first kidney transplant in 1966 and pioneered heart transplantation in 1967, SSA lags behind the developed world in transplant activity. According to WHO, SSA contributes the least number of transplant activity per WHO World region. Cost of treatment, low GDP, inadequate infrastructural and institutional support, dearth of facilities and technical expertise and absence of subsidy have all adversely affected organ donation and transplantation.

The health-care systems in SSA are weak and deficient. Peoples' decision to access healthcare services is influenced by knowledge of the disease condition, accessibility to health-care facility, affordability, religious and trado-cultural practices. Many people in LRCs patronize alternative healthcare service including traditional health providers and religious institutions as first choice resulting in late presentation to hospitals.

These challenges can be surmounted by adopting the 2007 World Health Organization Regional Consultation recommendations of establishment of national legal framework, self-sufficient organ donation and transplantation in each country, transparent transplantation practice, and prevention of commercialized transplantation and TT. In addition, establishment of national registries of organ transplantation is essential.

Author details

Ifeoma Ulasi[1,2,3]*, Chinwuba Ijoma[1,2], Ngozi Ifebunandu[3], Ejikeme Arodiwe[1,2], Uchenna Ijoma[1,2], Julius Okoye[2], Ugochi Onu[2], Chimezie Okwuonu[4], Sani Alhassan[5,6] and Obinna Onodugo[1,2]

1 College of Medicine, University of Nigeria, Ituku-Ozalla, Nigeria

2 University of Nigeria Teaching Hospital, Ituku-Ozalla, Enugu State, Nigeria

3 Alex Ekwueme Federal Teaching Hospital, Abakaliki, Ebonyi State, Nigeria

4 Federal Medical Centre, Umuahia, Abia State, Nigeria

5 Amino Kano Teaching Hospital, Kano, Nigeria

6 Bayero University, Kano, Nigeria

*Address all correspondence to: ifeoma.ulasi@unn.edu.ng

IntechOpen

© 2020 The Author(s). Licensee IntechOpen. This chapter is distributed under the terms of the Creative Commons Attribution License (http://creativecommons.org/licenses/by/3.0), which permits unrestricted use, distribution, and reproduction in any medium, provided the original work is properly cited. (cc) BY

References

[1] Freeman KJ. Transplant Program Personnel, Organization, and Function. In: Dunn SP, Horslen S, editors. Solid Organ Transplantation in Infants and Children, Organ and Tissue Transplantation, Springer International Publishing Switzerland; 2016. p. 1-13. DOI 10.1007/978-3-319-08049-9_4-1.

[2] Kaze AD, Ilori T, Jaar BG, Echouffo-Tcheugui JB. Burden of chronic kidney disease on the African continent: a systematic review and meta-analysis. BMC Nephrology. 2018;**19**:125 https://doi.org/10.1186/s12882-018-0930-5

[3] Loua A, Feroleto M, Sougou A, Kasilo OMJ, Nikiema JB, Fuller W, et al. A review of policies and programmes for human organ and tissue donations and transplantations, WHO African Region. *Bulletin of the World Health Organization* 2020;98:420-425. doi: http://dx.doi.org/10.2471/BLT.19.236992

[4] Dalal S, Beunza JJ, Volmink J, Adebamowo C, Bajunirwe F, Njelekela M, et al. Non-communicable diseases in sub-Saharan Africa: what we know now. International Journal of Epidemiology. 2011;**40**:885-890. DOI: 10.1093/ije/dyr050

[5] World health statistics 2018: monitoring health for the SDGs, sustainable development goals. Geneva: World Health Organization; 2018. Licence: CC BY-NC-SA 3.0 IGO. (Internet). 2018 Available from https://www.who.int/docs/default-source/gho-documents/world-health-statistic-reports/6-june-18108-world-health-statistics-2018.pdf (Accessed 10th September 2020).

[6] World Health Organization. The Double Burden: Emerging Epidemics and Persistent Problems. (Internet). Available From https://www.who.int/whr/1999/en/whr99_ch2_en.pdf?ua=1 (Accessed 10th September 2020).

[7] Stanifer JW, Jing B, Tolan S, Helmke N, Mukerjee R, Naicker S, et al. The epidemiology of chronic kidney disease in sub-Saharan Africa: a systematic review and meta-analysis. Lancet Glob Health. 2014;**2**:e174-e181 http://dx.doi.org/10.1016/S2214-109X(14)70002-6

[8] Atkins RC. The epidemiology of chronic kidney disease. *Kidney International*, Vol. 67, Supplement 94 (2005), pp. S14–S18.

[9] Abd ElHafeez S, Bolignano D, D'Arrigo G, Dounousi E, Tripepi G, Zoccali C. Prevalence and burden of chronic kidney disease among the general population and high-risk groups in Africa: a systematic review. BMJ Open. 2018;**8**:e015069. DOI: 10.1136/bmjopen-2016-015069

[10] HIV/AIDs: Key Facts. (Internet). 2020. Available from: https://www.who.int/news-room/fact-sheets/detail/hiv-aids (Accessed 20th September 2020).

[11] UNAIDS Fact Sheet. (Internet). 2020. Available from: https://www.unaids.org/sites/default/files/media_asset/UNAIDS_FactSheet_en.pdf (Accessed 20th September 2020).

[12] Benedetti C, Waldman M, Zaza G, Riella LV and Cravedi P (2020) COVID-19 and the Kidneys: An Update. Front. Med. 7:423. doi: 10.3389/fmed.2020.00423

[13] WHO. New hepatitis data highlight need for urgent global response. (Internet). 2017. Available from: https://www.who.int/news-room/detail/21-04-2017-new-hepatitis-data-highlight-need-for-urgent-global-response (Accessed 20th September 2020)

[14] Fattovich G, Guistina G, Degos F, Tremolada F, Diodati G, Almasio P. Morbidity and mortality in

compensated cirrhosis type C: A retrospective follow-up study of 384 patients. Gastroenterology. 1997;**112**:463-472

[15] Kim WR, Thermeau TM, Benson JT, Kremers WK, Rosen CB, Gores GJ, et al. Deaths on the liver transplant waiting list:An analysis of competing risks. Hepatology. 2006;**43**:345-351

[16] Mahillo B, Carmona M, Alvarez M, Marco J, Nuñez JR, López-Fraga M, et al. Worldwide distribution of solid organ transplantation and access of population to those practices. Transplantation. 2018;**102**:7S

[17] GODT. International Report on Organ Donation and Transplantation Activities Executive summary 2017. (Internet). 2017. Available from: http://www.transplant-observatory.org/ (Accessed 10th September 2020).

[18] World Bank Data. Population, total - Sub-Saharan Africa. (Internet). 2019. Available from: https://data.worldbank.org/indicator/SP.POP.TOTL?locations=ZG (Accessed 20th September 2020)

[19] United Nations, Department of Economic and Social Affairs, Population Division (2019). *World Population Prospects 2019: Data Booklet* (ST/ESA/SER.A/424). (Internet). 2019. Available from. https://population.un.org/wpp/Publications/Files/WPP2019_DataBooklet (Accessed 24th September 2020)

[20] Kobayashi S, Hidaka S. Can we still ignore renal replacement therapy in sub-Saharan Africa? All living beings are created equal. (2020) 6:5 https://doi.org/10.1186/s41100-019-0243-6

[21] World Health Organization (WHO). Everybody's business: Strengthening health systems to improve health outcomes-WHO's framework for action. 2007. Geneva: WHO

[22] Ayanore MA, Amuna N, Aviisah M, Awolu A, Kipo-Sunyehzi DD, Mogre V, et al.., 2019. Towards Resilient Health Systems in Sub-Saharan Africa: A Systematic Review of the English Language Literature on Health Workforce, Surveillance, and Health Governance Issues for Health Systems Strengthening. *Annals of Global Health* 2019: 85(1), p.113. DOI: http://doi.org/10.5334/aogh.2514

[23] Aldis W. Health security as a public health concept: A critical analysis. *Health Policy and Planning*. 2008; 23: 369-375. DOI: https://doi.org/10.1093/heapol/czn030

[24] Ojong N. The COVID-19 Pandemic and the Pathology of the Economic and Political Architecture in Cameroon. *Healthcare* 2020; *8*: 176; doi:10.3390/healthcare8020176

[25] Bryan L, Conway M, Keesmaat T, McKenna S, Richardson B. A practical approach to health system strengthening in sub-Saharan Africa. Health International 2009; 9: 80 – 95. (Internet). Available from: https://www.mckinsey.com/~/media/mckinsey/dotcom/client_service/Healthcare%20Systems%20and%20Services/Health%20International/HI09_Africa.ashx (Accessed 24th September 2020).

[26] Jacobs B, Ir P, Bigdeli M, Annear PL, Damme WV. Addressing access barriers to health services: an analytical framework for selecting appropriate interventions in low-income Asian countries. Health Policy and Planning 2011; 1-13 doi:10.1093/heapol/czr038.

[27] Ulasi II, Ijoma CK. The enormity of chronic kidney disease in Nigeria: the situation in a teaching hospital in South-east Nigeria. *Journal of Tropical Medicine 2010.* 2010, Article ID 501957, 6 pages. doi:10.1155/2010/501957;2010.

[28] African Economic Outlook 2020. (Internet). 2020. Available from:

https://www.afdb.org/en/knowledge/publications/african-economic-outlook (Accessed 2oth September 2020).

[29] African Economic Outlook 2020 Supplement Amid COVID-19. (Internet). 2020. Available from: https://dataportal.opendataforafrica.org/wozrhgf/african-economic-outlook-supplement-amid-covid-19 (Accessed 2oth September 2020).

[30] Jowett M, Brunal MP, Flores G, Cylus J. Spending targets for health: no magic number. Geneva: World Health Organization; 2016 (WHO/HIS/HGF/HFWorkingPaper/16.1; Health Financing Working Paper No. 1); http://apps.who.int/iris/bitstream/10665/250048/1/WHO-HIS-HGF- HFWorkingPaper-16.1-eng.pdf

[31] World Health Organization, Public financing for health in Africa: from Abuja to the SDGs. 2016, WHO: Geneva.

[32] Atlas of African Health Statistics 2018: universal health coverage and the Sustainable Development Goals in the WHO African Region. Brazzaville: WHO Regional Office for Africa; 2018. Licence: CC BY-NC-SA 3.0 IGO.

[33] Fabian J, Maher H, Bentley A, Gaylard P, Crymble K, Rossi B et al. Favourable outcomes for the first 10 years of kidney and pancreas transplantation at Wits Donald Gordon Medical Centre, Johannesburg, South Africa. S Afr Med J 2016;106(2):172-176. https://doi.org/10.7196/SAMJ.2016.v106i2.10190

[34] Brink JG, Hassoulas J. The first human heart transplant and further advances in cardiac transplantation at groote schuur hospital and the University of Cape town. *Cardiovasc J Afr* 2009; 20: 31-35.

[35] Moosa MR. The state of kidney transplantation in South Africa. S Afr Med J 2019;109(4):235-240. DOI:10.7196/SAMJ.2019.v109i4.13548

[36] Delmonico FL, Domínguez-Gil B, Matesanz R,Noel L. A call for government accountability to achieve national self-sufficiency in organ donation and transplantation. Lancet 2011; 378(9800): 1414-1418. https://doi.org/10.1016/S0140-6736(11)61486-4

[37] Muller E. Organ donation and transplantation in South Africa – an update. Continuing Medical Education 2013; 31 (6). http://www.cmej.org.za/index.php/cmej/rt/printerFriendly/2764/3004

[38] Muller E, Kahn D, Mendelson M. Renal transplantation between HIV-positive donor and recipients. N Engl J Med 2010; 362(24): 2336-2337.

[39] Muller E, Barday Z. HIV-Positive Kidney Donor Selection for HIV-Positive Transplant Recipients. J Am Soc Nephrol. 2018 Apr; 29(4): 1090-1095. doi: 10.1681/ASN.2017080853.

[40] Bento I. First-ever kidney transplant in Namibia a success. (Internet). 2016. Available from: https://www.nampa.org/index.php?model=feature&function=display&id=124269 (Accessed 26th September 2020).

[41] WHO: Regional Committee for Africa. Status of Human Organ and Tissue Donation and Transplantation in the Who African Region. Report of the Secretariat AFR/RC70/12 30 June 2020. (Internet). 2020. Available from: https://www.afro.who.int/sites/default/files/2020-07/AFR-RC70-12%20Status%20of%20human%20organ%20and%20tissue%20donation%20and%20transplantation.pdf (Accessed 10th October 2020).

[42] Osafo C, Morton B, Ready A, Jewett-Harris, Adu D. Organ Transplantation in Ghana. Transplantation 2018: 102 (4): 539 – 541.

[43] Lagou DA, Ackoundou-N'guessan KC, Njapom TL, Sekongo YM, Guei CM, Tia MW. Characteristics and Outcome of Living Kidney Donors After Donation: A Report from Cote d'Ivoire. Saudi J Kidney Dis Transpl 2016;27(3):563-568.

[44] Ackoundou-N'Guessan C, Hoang AD, Ben Abdallah T, Gnionsahe DA, Dollo I, Ripoche C, et al. Living Kidney Donor Transplantation in a Resource-limited Country: The Ivory Coast Experience. Transplant Proc. Jul-Aug 2015;47(6):1580-4. doi: 10.1016/j.transproceed.2015.03.053.

[45] Ulasi II, Ijoma CK. Organ Transplantation in Nigeria. Transplantation ! April 2016; 100 (4): 695 -697.

[46] Ahmed MM, Tedla FM, Leichtman AB, Punch JD. Organ Transplantation in Ethiopia. Transplantation 2019; 103 (3): 449 – 451.

[47] Ministry of Health, Kenya. 10 years and 200 transplants later! KNH celebrates a milestone. (Internet) 2019. Available from: https://www.health.go.ke/10-years-and-200-transplants-later-knh-celebrates-a-milestone/ (Accessed 23rd September 2020).

[48] The Evolution of Renal Transplantation in Mauritius (1980 – 1997). Transplant Int 2001; 14: 115 – 116.

[49] Gopee N. The Renal Transplantation issue. (Internet) 2018. Available from: http://www.mauritiustimes.com/mt/the-renal-transplantation-issue/ (Accessed 23rd September 2020).

[50] Ahmed IAM, Musa EA, Shaikh Q, Elsharif ME. Kidney Transplantation in Sudan. Transplantation 2018; 102 (10): 1583 – 1585.

[51] Furia FF, Shoo J, Ruggajo PJ, Kilonzo K, Basu G, Yeates K, et al. Developing nephrology services in low income countries: a case of Tanzania. BMC Nephrology (2019) 20:378 https://doi.org/10.1186/s12882-019-1568-7

[52] Kazibwe K. Cabinet approves bill that allows body organ donation, transplant. (Internet). 2020 Available from: https://nilepost.co.ug/2020/06/07/cabinet-approves-bill-that-allows-body-organ-donation-transplant/ (Accessed 23rd September 2020).

[53] Jahora R. Angola Paves the Way for Organ Transplants. (Internet) 2019. Available from: http://www.ahora.cu/en/sport/15-section/world/4740-angola-paves-the-way-for-organ-transplants (Accessed 24th September 2020).

[54] Ulasi I, Ijoma C, Onodugo O, Arodiwe E, Okoye J, Onu U, et al. Posttransplant care of kidney transplant recipients and their donors in Nigeria. Exp Clin Transplant 2019; 17 (Suppl 1): 50 – 56.

[55] KDIGO Clinical Practice Guideline on the Evaluation and Management of Candidates for Kidney Transplantation. *Transplantation* 2020;104: S1–S103

[56] Renal Association Clinical Practice Guideline on the Assessment of the Potential Kidney Transplant Recipient. Nephron Clinical Practice 2011;118 Suppl 1(Suppl. 1):c209-24

[57] Knoll G, Cockfield S, Blydt-Hansen T, Baran D, Kiberd B, Landsberg D et al. Canadian Society of Transplantation: consensus guidelines on eligibility for kidney transplantation. CMAJ : Canadian Medical Association Journal = Journal de L'association Medicale Canadienne. 2005 Nov;173(10):S1-25. DOI: 10.1503/cmaj.1041588.

[58] Dye C, Scheeles S, Dominic P, et al. Global burden of tuberculosis: Estimated incidence, prevalence and

morbidity by country. JAMA 1999; 282: 677-686.

[59] Ghods A J. Living kidney donation: The outcomes for donors. Int J Organ Transplant Med 2010; 1(2): 63-71.

[60] Fehrman-Ekholn I, Elinder CG, Stenbeck M, et al. Kidney donors live longer. Transplantation 1997; 64: 976-978.

[61] Ibrahim HN, Foley R, Tan LP, et al. Long term consequences of kidney donation. N Engl J Med 2009; 360:459-469.

[62] Organ Procurement and Transplantation Network Living Donor Committee: Living donation. Available from. http://optn.transplant.hrsa.gov/ Policies and Byelaws2/policies/pdf/ policy .

[63] House RM 1993. Cited in Erick M, Christine E Skotzko CE. Psychiatric assessment in transplantation Rev. Saúde Pública, 34 (4): 415-20, 2000 www.fsp.usp.br/rsp.

[64] Castelnuovo TP (1981) "Transplantation: psychological implications of changes in body image" in Psychonephrology. Psychological factors in hemodialysis and trasplantion; Levy (Ed). Plenum Press, New York.

[65] De Baere C, Delva D, Kloeck A, et al. Return to work and social participation: does type of organ transplantation matter? Transplantation. 2010;89(8):1009-1015.

[66] Van der Mei SF, Krol B, van Son WJ, de Jong PE, Groothoff JW, van den Heuvel WJ. Social participation and employment status after kidney transplantation: a systematic review. Qual Life Res. 2006;15(6):979-994.

[67] Paris W, White-Williams C. Social adaptation after cardiothoracic transplantation: a review of the literature. J Cardiovasc Nurs. 2005; 20(5 Suppl):S67–S73.

[68] Huda A, Newcomer R, Harrington C, Keeffe EB, Esquivel CO. Employment after liver transplantation: a review. Transplant Proc. 2015;47(2):233-239.

[69] Mata AJ, Garvey CA, Jacobs CL, Kahn JP. Non-directed donation of kidneys from living donors. New Engl J Med 2000, 343(6), 433-436.

[70] Simmons RG, Marine SK, Simmons RLSimmons RG. Gift of life: The social and psychological impact of organ transplantation. NY: Wiley, 1977. Reprinted with additions, Brunswick, NJ: Transaction Books,1987.

[71] Goetzmann L, Irani S, Moser KS, Schwegler K, Stamm M, Spindler A, et al. Goetzmann Psychological processing of transplantation in lung recipients: a quantitative study of organ integration and the relationship to the donor. Br J Health Psychol. 2009; 14(pt 4):667-680.

[72] Heinrich TW, Marcangelo M. Psychiatric issues in solid organ transplantation. Harv Rev Psychiatry. 2009;17(6):398-406.

[73] Smith GC, Trauer T, Kerr PG, Chadban SJ. Prospective psychosocial monitoring of living kidney donors using the Short Form-36 Health Survey: Results at 12 months. Transplantation 2004, 78(9), 1384-1389.

[74] Olbrisch ME, Benedict SM, Cropsey KL. Psychological, social and behavioral characteristics of living donor candidates for adult liver transplantation. Biennial meeting on Psychiatric, Psychosocial and Ethical Issues in Organ Transplantation, February, 2005, Santa Monica, CA.

[75] Hirvas J, Enckell M, Kuhlback B, Pasternack A. Psychological and social

problems encountered in active treatments of chronic uraemia. The living donor. ActaMedicaScandinavica, 1976, 200, 17-20.

[76] Simmons RG, Anderson CR. Related donors and recipients: five to nine years post-transplant. Transplant Proc 1982, 14, 9-12.

[77] Simmons RG. Related donors: Costs and gains. Transplant Proc 1977, 9, 143-145.

[78] Chevrollier GS, McCune K, Sha AP, Live Donor Nephrectomy; Contemporary Kidney Transplantation pp1-21, Organ and Tissue Transplantation Springer International Publishing AG, part of Springer Nature 2018 C.G.B. Ramirez, J. McCauley (eds.).

[79] Doria C, Margetich L; Recipient Renal Transplantation pp1-11, Contemporary Kidney Transplantation pp1-21, Organ and Tissue Transplantation Springer International Publishing AG, part of Springer Nature 2018 C.G.B. Ramirez, J. McCauley (eds.)

[80] McCauley J,A History of Kidney Transplantation, Contemporary Kidney Transplantation pp1-23, Organ and Tissue Transplantation Springer International Publishing AG, part of Springer Nature 2018 C.G.B. Ramirez, J. McCauley (eds.)

[81] Kasiske BL,Cangro CB, Hariharan S et al. The evaluation of renal transplant candidates: clinical practice guidelines. Am J Transplant 2001;1 [Suppl 2]:1-95.

[82] Khan T, Kamal S, Koshaji B, et al. Delayed graft function in living donor kidney transplantation. Ann Transplant, 2013;18:434-5.

[83] Davidson B, Du Toit T, Jones ESW, Barday Z, Manning K, Curdie F, et al. (2019) Outcomes and challenges of a kidney transplant programme at Groote Schuur Hospital, Cape Town: A South African perspective. *PLOS ONE* 14(1): e0211189. https://doi.org/10.1371/journal.pone.0211189

[84] Bakari AA, Jimeta USA, Abubakar MA, Alhassan SU, Nwankwo EA. Organ Transplantation: Legal, Ethical and Islamic Perspective in Nigeria. Nigerian Journal of Surgery 2012; 18 (2): 53 – 60.

[85] Boima V, Ganu V, Dey V, Yorke E, Yawson A, Otchere Y, et al. Kidney transplantation in Ghana; Is the public ready? Clin Transplant 2017; 31(10). doi: 10.1111/ctr.13061.

[86] Kim I, Noh H, Ji E, Hong SH, Ha J, Burckart et. al.Identification of factors affecting tacrolimus level and 5- year clinical outcome in kidney transplant patients. Basic clin pharmacol toxicol 2012;111:217-223 https://doi.org/10.1111/j.1742-7843.2012.00892.x

[87] Hu RH, Lee PH, Tsai MK. Clinical influencing factors for daily dose, trough level, and relative clearance of tacrolimus in renal transplant recipients. Transplant Proc 2000;32: 1689-1692.

[88] Fitzsimmons WE, Bekersky I, Dressler D, Raye K, Hodosh E, Mekki Q. Demographic considerations in tacrolimus pharmacokinetics. Transplant Proc. 1998;30: 1359-1364.

[89] Braun F, Schütz E, Christians U, Lorf T, Schiffmann JH, Armstrong VW, et al. Pitfalls in monitoring tacrolimus (FK 506). Ther Drug Monit 1997;19:628-31.

[90] Dirks NL, Huth B, Yates CR, Meibohm B. Pharmacokinetics of immunosuppressants: a perspective on ethnic differences. International journal of clinical pharmacology and therapeutics 2004;42:701-718.

[91] Neylan, JF. Racial differences in renal transplantation after immunosuppression with tacrolimus versus cyclosporine. FK506 Kidney Transplant Study Group. Transplantation 1998;65:515-23.

[92] Leichtman AB, Cohen D, Keith D, O'Connor KO, Goldstein M, McBride V. et al. Kidney and pancreas transplantation in the United States,1997-2006: the HRSA Breakthrough Collaboratives and the 58 DSA Challenge. Am J Transplant, 2008 8(Part 2): 946 – 957.

[93] Muller E, White SL, Delmonico F. Regional perspective; Developing organ transplantation in Sub-Saharan Africa. Transplantation 2014, 97(10): 975-976.

[94] World Bank. Poverty and Equity Brief – Sub Saharan Africa. (Internet). 2020. Available from: https://databank.worldbank.org/data/download/poverty/33EF03BB-9722-4AE2-ABC7-AA2972D68AFE/Global_POVEQ_SSA.pdf (Accessed 10th October 2020).

[95] Arogundade FA. Kidney transplantation in a low-resource setting: Nigeria experience. Kidney Int Suppl (2013) 3:241-245.

[96] Sub-Saharan Africa Unemployment Rate 1991-2020. (Internet). 2020. Available from: https://www.macrotrends.net/countries/SSF/sub-saharan-africa-/unemployment-rate (Accessed 10th October 2020).

[97] The declaration of Istanbul on organ trafficking and transplant tourism. Kidney International (2008) 74, 854-859; doi:10.1038/ki.2008.388.

[98] O'Connell PJ, Brown M, Chan TM, Granado RC, Davies SJ, Eiam-Ong S *et. al*. The role of kidney transplantation as a component of integrated care for chronic kidney disease. Kidney International Supplements (2020) 10, e78–e85; https://doi.org/10.1016/j.kisu.2019.11.006

[99] Lavee J, Ashkenazi T, Stoler A, Cohen J, Beyar R. Preliminary marked increase in the national organ donation rate in Israel following implementation of a new organ transplantation law. Am J Transplant 2013;13(3):780-785. https://doi.org/10.1111/ajt.12001

[100] Lavee J, Brock DW. Prioritizing registered donors in organ allocation: an ethical appraisal of the Israeli organ transplant law. Curr Opin Crit Care 2012, 18:000-000. DOI:10.1097/MCC.0b013e328357a2e2

[101] Akoh JA. Renal transplantation in developing countries. Saudi J Kidney Dis Transpl 2011;22(4):637-650.

[102] Chugh KS, Jha V. Problems and outcomes of living unrelated donor transplants in the developing countries. Kidney Int 2000;57: S131-5.

[103] Rizvi A, Naqvi A. Need for increasing transplant activity: A sustainable model for developing countries. Transplant Proc 1997; 29:1560-1562.

[104] Rizvi SAH, Naqvi SAA, Zafar MN et al: A Renal Transplantation Model for developing countries. Am J Transplant 2011: 11: 2302-2307.

[105] Ghods AJ, Savaj S. Iranian Model of Paid and Regulated Living-Unrelated Kidney Donation. *Clin J Am Soc Nephrol* 1: 1136-1145, 2006. doi: 10.2215/CJN.00700206

[106] WHA57/18. Human organ and tissue transplantation. In: Fifty-seventh World Health Assembly, Geneva, 17-22 May 2004. Resolutions and Decisions. Geneva: World Health Organization; 2010. (Internet). Available from: https://apps.who.int/gb/ebwha/pdf_files/WHA57/A57_R18-en.pdf (Accessed 23rd September).

[107] WHA63/22. Human organ and tissue transplantation. In: Sixty-third World Health Assembly, Geneva, 17-21 May 2010. Geneva: World Health Organization; 2010. (Internet). Available from: https://apps.who.int/gb/ebwha/pdf_files/WHA63/A63_R22-en.pdf?ua=1 (Accessed 23rd September).

[108] WHO Guiding Principles on human cell, tissue and organ transplantation. Geneva: World Health Organization; 2010. (Internet). Available from: https://www.who.int/transplantation/Guiding_principlestransplantation_WHA63.22en.pdf?Ua=1 (Accessed 29th September 2020).

[109] United Nations General Assembly Resolution 71/322. Strengthening and promoting effective measures and international cooperation on organ donation and transplantation to prevent and combat trafficking in persons for the purpose of organ removal and trafficking in human organs. 2017 (Internet) Available from: https://undocs.org/pdf?symbol=en/A/RES/71/322 (Accessed 29th September 2020).

[110] WHO Task Force on Donation and Transplantation of Human Organs and Tissues. 2017 (). Available from: https://www.who.int/transplantation/donation/taskforce-transplantation/en/ (Accessed 29th September 2020).

[111] Davids MR, Eastwood JB, Selwood NH, Arogundade FA, Ashuntantang G, Benghanem Gharbi M, et al. A renal registry for Africa: first steps. Clinical Kidney Journal, vol. 9, no. 1, 162-167; 2016

Section 2

Organ Procurement

Chapter 3

Surgical Techniques of Multiorgan Procurement from a Deceased Donor

Farzad Kakaei

Abstract

Solid organ transplantation is now the standard treatment for many types of diseases and using a standard surgical technique for organ procurement from the deceased donors is an important step in preventing complications after such complicated procedures. In most centers, retrieval of heart, lungs, liver, kidneys, small bowel, pancreas and other organs is done at the same time by different surgeons under supervision by a team leader who is most familiar with at least basic steps of surgical technique of procurement of all the solid organs. Each transplant surgeon, regardless of his or her sub-specialty, has to know how to prepare and dissect the delicate anatomical structures which are in common between the two adjacent organs for example portal vein (liver-pancreas), superior mesenteric vein (pancreas-small bowel), abdominal inferior vena cava (liver-kidneys), supra-diaphragmatic inferior vena cava (liver-heart) and pulmonary artery-veins (heart-lungs). This needs a multidisciplinary approach by the most experienced members of the transplant team to decrease the warm ischemic time of the organs without any harm to them by better coordination between all the surgeons. In this, chapter we briefly describe the multiorgan retrieval procedure in a deceased donor, and we hope that following these instructions results in better quality of the procured organs without jeopardizing their vital anatomical structures.

Keywords: organ transplantation, multiorgan procurement, deceased donor, surgery, technique

1. Introduction

Organ transplantation from deceased donor is the standard technique for treatment of so many diseases which is totally incurable without such complicated surgeries. A deceased donor has multiple solid organs that may be used for transplantation and multidisciplinary approach and delicate coordination between different medical and surgical teams is needed to ensure that these organs are fully functional after retrieval. Heart, lungs, liver, kidneys, pancreas and small bowel are among the most important organs that should be harvested at the same time from one donor and each surgeon who is in charge of such a complicated surgery should be familiar with at least basic techniques of other organs retrieval to prevent any harm to sensitive anatomic components of each organ especially those which are in common between two nearby organs, for example portal vein and celiac trunk (liver and pancreas), abdominal inferior vena cava (liver and kidneys), superior mesenteric artery and vein (pancreas and small intestine), supra-diaphragmatic inferior vena cava (heart and liver), pulmonary artery and veins (heart and lungs). Chairman of the team should be the most expert surgeon who has the longest experience with all aspects of multiorgan procurement surgery. In this chapter we will be discuss the basic aspects of surgical techniques which every transplant surgeon has to know about such an important procedure.

2. Brief history of multiorgan donation

The era of organ transplantation was started successful kidney transplantation in the early 1950s. First organ donation from non-heart-beating donors was associated with successful liver transplantation by Thomas Starzl in 1963 [1]. First rare heart-beating donors without any hope of survival (not living donors) were those who underwent cardiac bypass but not able to detach from the heart-lung machine whose kidneys were used for transplantation before death in 1962 [2]. Next successful transplantation from heart-beating donors were done in 1964 in Sweden and in 1966 in United States from patients with irreversible brain damage under mechanical ventilation [2]. The term "cerebral death" was supposed by Swedish neurosurgeons in 1965 [3]. First series of successful liver transplantations from such "brain death" donors was done by Thomas Starzl in 1967–1968 and Professor Barnard do the first successful heart transplant in the same year from another brain-dead person [2]. At that time Barnard waited for cardiac asystole to prevent any negative debate for "brain death concept" in the community [4]. In the next decade many authorities in all the pioneer countries in transplantation made every effort to legally confirm the brain death patients as a potential donor and at last in 1971 the "Uniform Anatomical Gift Act" in Kansas was approved by the governor as a basis for globalization of legally "brain death concept" [5]. Development of multiple transplant teams in next decade resulted in first multiorgan retrieval procedures from the same donor in the 1980s [6, 7]. First heart-lung transplant was done in 1982 and first long term survived lung transplant alone was done in 1987 [8]. In the same era till the 1990s, successful combined transplantation such as liver combined with small bowel and other more complex multivisceral transplantation was developed by Thomas Starzl and his former fellow Andreas Tzakis [9]. Thanks to all the pioneers' efforts, now we have a near standard technique for multiorgan procurement from all stable brain-dead donors. Only the availability of all the team members and also the suitability of all the organs and suitable recipients are among the remaining obstacle such a complex procedure and multiorgan donation at the same time is a rule in most experienced transplant centers.

3. Donor management

Ideally, every deceased donor should be completely stable before and during transfer to the operating theater. Central venous pressure should be maintained between 10 and 12 mmHg for better function of abdominal organs but for lung retrieval this pressure should be maintained around 8 mmHg [10]. Systolic blood pressure maintenance over 100 mmHg and mean arterial pressure over 60 mmHg by using inotropes and crystalloid infusion is critical. Dopamine, dobutamine, vasopressin and nor-adrenaline may be used but when heart is being used for transplantation dosage of nor-adrenaline over 0.05 microgram/kg/min may reduce cardiac contractility after transplantation and should be avoided [11]. In such cases insertion of Swan-Ganz catheter is mandatory.

Every effort should be done to maintain PaO_2 > 100 mmHg, SpO_2 > 95%, $PaCO_2$ between 35 and 40 mmHg and pH between 7.35 and 7.45 by using lung protective strategy including avoidance of excessive intravenous fluids, minimal tidal volume (8–12/minute) and lowest FiO_2 [12].

For hormonal management, intravenous infusion of 1000 mg (15 mg/kg) methylprednisolone succinate, insulin (target glucose level of 80–150 mg/dl), vasopressin 0.5–4 U/h) or intranasal desmopressin (1–2 puff every 6 hours) and thyroxine replacement (4 mcg/h) is the standard of treatment to reduce the systemic inflammatory response in these patients and maintaining the hemodynamic stability of them [10].

Urine output is better maintained between 100 and 300 ml/hour to prevent hypo or hypernatremia. Potassium (K^+) replacement should be started when serum potassium level is reduced (target K^+ level 3.5–4.5 meq/l). Lactated ringer's solution or half saline solution is the best available fluid for these patients and using colloids such as albumin should be avoided [13].

Body temperature should be maintained over 35.8°C [13] for better cardiac function and prevention of coagulation cascade and hypoxic tissue damage. To reduce cardiac arrhythmias maintaining normal body temperature, hemodynamics, electrolyte, hemoglobin levels over 10 g/dl and minimal use of vasopressors is essential. Calcium, phosphorus and magnesium also should be maintained at physiologic level to prevent cardiac arrhythmias during the surgery [14].

4. Key controversies in the result of multiorgan procurement

We have many unresolved issues about multiorgan procurement surgery that needs more time to answer by the researchers. As the same with other works which are done by a team, expertise of each of the team member and their coordination with other members have a great effect on the final result of the operation. Undoubtedly, multiorgan retrieval may compromise the function of each organ and will be associated with a higher incidence of delicate anatomical structures damage. It may be better to perform all the dissections without any compromise in the circulation of any other organs. Many researchers show that this concern is not completely definite. Even some authors in their prospective and retrospective studies show that multiorgan harvesting may improve each separate organ function [10]. The main factor that affects the final result is the stability of the patient during the operation and the expertise of who is in charge of the whole operation [15]. One study shows that renal anatomical damage is more common when the operation is done by renal team only and if the operation is done by the liver team with experience of more than 50 procurement per year, the final anatomical (artery, vein ureter or capsular) damage will be significantly reduced [16]. In unstable patients, it is the duty of the team leader to determine which organ is more important and is the first priority. Usually in urgent situations, this is the "liver", because liver transplantation has the only way to cure the hepatic failure without any other treatment option in these patients with an acceptable success rate.

Another concern is that should dissection be done in warm or cold condition and en-bloc or separate organ retrieval is different? In fact, although theoretically the anatomical damage may be reduced if all the delicate dissections are performed in the donor before clamping of the aorta and all the organs retrieved separately, but most studies show that en-bloc retrieval and continuing the dissections after whole body cooling and whole blood evacuation have better results [10]. The rationale for this concept is that complete dissection especially in inexperienced hands is extremely time consuming and may result in end organ ischemia by inducing vasospasm. Using rapid technique is more acceptable for operating room personnel and other members of the team, and this technique that one was used only for unstable donors is now the routine in most transplant centers [10].

Although most centers are reluctant to change their previous successful policies and it is a routine to perform double cannulation (aortic and portal) for dual perfusion of the liver, but nowadays with increased use of the pancreas and small bowel for transplantation, double perfusion may be replaced by the single aortic perfusion as a rule for most deceased donors [10]. With the advent of machine perfusion which used only one system for ex situ perfusion, there is increasingly more doubt about need for double perfusion and most studies shows that arterial perfusion is more important in saving the organ function especially the biliary system [17].

5. Type, volume, and pressure of preservation solution

Historically, blood is the first perfusate that was used for organ preservation [18]. After that, Alexis Carrel reported the first nOn-bood solution named Tyrode's solution which can preserve cat thyroid tissue viable for 3–21 days [18]. In 1960s hypothermia added to blood or serum for better survival of kidney grafts. Since then, static cold storage (STS) by perfusion of the organs by cold (0–4°C) solutions was accepted as the gold standard for organ preservation till now [18]. Collin's solution (invented in 1969) and then Euro-Collin's (1980) were the standard solution for organ preservation for next two decades and at last University of Wisconsin (UW) solution was invented by Belzer in 1985 [19]. This solution is low Na^+, high K^+ solution like intracellular fluid (ICF) which was the gold standard for organ preservation for at least 2 decades.

Histidine-tryptophan-ketoglutarate (HTK) (low Na^+, high K^+ with cardioplegic effects) and Celsior (high Na^+, low K^+) solutions are next preservative fluids which was initially used only for heart transplantation in 1990s which were much cheaper and very soon, UW was replaced by these solutions in all abdominal organ transplantations in some transplant centers [18]. Although, these solutions have lower cost and lower viscosities, but till now, UW is the standard solution for heart transplantation in most centers [20]. IGL-1® (Institute George Lopez-1) liquid is another low viscosity solution which reversed electrolyte concentration compared with UW (K+ 25 meq/l, Na + 120 meq/l) with lower cardiac complication and some centers proved that with the use of this liquid, the results of liver and kidney transplantation will be better.

High K^+ concentration of this solution made them unsuitable for lung transplantation because of high risk of pulmonary vasoconstriction [20]. Perfadex® (a low-potassium dextran glucose solution) was invented with characteristics of extracellular fluid for this purpose in late 1980s and since then then is used as the standard preservative for lung transplantation [18].

In multiorgan procurement procedure which is a routine procedure in high volume transplant centers, each team usually used its preferred solution for individual organ transplantation. For example, cardiac and abdominal teams may choose HTK or UW solution but pulmonary team uses Perfadex®, and when a heart-lung transplantation is performed en-bloc in one person, then they should use a cardioplegic solution first and after that Perfadex® for pulmonary preservation. **Table 1** shows the characteristics of most popular different preservation solutions which are commercially available now.

Another dilemma that should be resolved is the rate and pressure of preservative solutions. Perfusion by a cold perfusate in not a physiologic process and most teams

Name of the solution	Osmolar characteristic	Major composition
Viaspan® (UW solution, University of Wisconsin solution)	Intracellular	K^+ 125 meq/l (prevents the K^+ transudation of the cells but may cause vasoconstriction) Na + 29 meq/l Hydroxyethyl starch (HES) (reduce extravasation of the fluids but by increasing the viscosity and RBC aggregation may increase renal damage) Raffinose (prevention of cell swelling after cooling) Glutathione (reduction of oxidative effects of free oxygen radicals) Adenosine (increase ATP levels) Allopurinol (protective effect in ischemia by xanthine oxidase inhibition) Lactobionic acid (prevention of intracellular edema)
HTK®	Extracellular	K^+ 9 meq/l Na^+ 15 meq/l Histidine (precursor for energy metabolism and buffering effect) Tryptophan (cell membrane stabilization and oxygen free radicals' removal) α-ketoglutaric acid (primary substrate for anaerobic metabolism) Mannitol (prevents hypothermic cell swelling) Higher volume is needed (6–10 lit) Diastolic cardiac arrest
IGL-1®	Extracellular	Based on UW with reversed Na^+/K^+ concentration (may reduce cardiovascular complication) K^+ 25 meq/l Na^+ 120 meq/l Polyethylene glycol (PEG-35) (instead of HES for stabilization of the lipid layer of the cell membrane) Allopurinol (protective effect in ischemia by xanthine oxidase inhibition) Adenosine (increase ATP levels) Raffinose (prevention of cell swelling after cooling) Glutathione (reduction of oxidative effects of free oxygen radicals)
Celsior®	Extracellular	K^+ 15 meq/l Na^+ 100 meq/l 320–360 mOsm/l (hypertonic) Lactobionic acid (prevention of intracellular edema) Mannitol (prevents hypothermic cell swelling) Histidine (precursor for energy metabolism and buffering effect) Glutathione (reduction of oxidative effects of free oxygen radicals) Glutamate (prevent intracellular flush of calcium)
Plegisol®	Extracellular	K^+ 16 meq/l Na^+ 110 meq/l Osmolarity of 328 mOsm/l and pH = 7.8. Ca^{2+} (for prevention of calcium flush and sarcolemmic cracking Phosphate buffer (counteracts the effects of metabolic acidosis). Mg^{2+} is (myocardial stabilization by inhibition of myosin chain phosphorylation) Suitable only for cardiac transplant

Name of the solution	Osmolar characteristic	Major composition
Polysol (PS)	Extracellular	Na^+ 120 meq/l K^+ 15 meq/l Osmolarity 320 mOsm/l. Polyethylene glycol (PEG-35) (stabilization of the lipid layer of the cell membrane) Phosphate buffer (counteracts the effects of metabolic acidosis). Histidine (precursor for energy metabolism and buffering effect HEPES (buffer of N-(2-hydroxyethyl) piperazine-N-2-ethanesulfonic acid) Glutathione (reduction of oxidative effects of free oxygen radicals) Raffinose (prevention of cell swelling after cooling) Trehalose (cytoprotective effect) Vitamins B1, B2, B3, B4, B5, B6, B7, B8, B9, B12, C, A, D2, E, and K3 21 amino acids (alanine, arginine, asparagine, cysteine, glutamine, glycine, isoleucine, leucine, lysine, methionine, ornithine, phenylalanine, proline, serine, threonine, tryptophan, tyrosine, valine)
Perfadex®	Extracellular	Na^+ 138 meq/lit K^+ 6 meq/l Osmolarity 292 mOsm/l pH 7.4) Dextran 40 (50 g/l) (maintains fluids in the endovascular space) Glucose (as a source of energy) Phosphate buffer (counteracts the effects of metabolic acidosis) Suitable only for lung preservation
ET-Kyoto	extracellular	Na^+ 107 mmol/l K^+ 42 meq/l Osmolarity 366 mOsm/l Trehalose (cytoprotective effect) Gluconate (counteract cell swelling) Hydroxyethyl starch (HES) (reduce extravasation of the fluids but by increasing the viscosity and RBC aggregation may increase renal damage) Phosphate buffer (prevents metabolic acidosis) Db-cAMP (cyclic adenosine monophosphate dibutyltin) Nitroglycerine (protect the vascular endothelial cells) N-acetylcysteine (NAC) (antioxidant effect and a free radical scavenger) Approved only for lung transplantation

Table 1.
Characteristics of different popular preservation solutions.

accepted the 80–100 cm H_2O (1 m gravity pressure) as the acceptable pressure for all organs and 150 cm H_2O for aortic infusion [10]. With the advent of machine perfusion, it is shown that target arterial flow of 0.25 mL/minute/g and target v0nous flow of 0.75 mL/minute/g liver tissue and mean arterial and portal venous pressure of 30–50 and 8–10 mmHg, respectively, are the acceptable rates for liver transplantation and these figures could be extrapolated to the multiple abdominal organ retrieval procedure [21]. Higher pressure for portal vein irrigation is definitively deleterious for post-transplant function of the graft. For pancreas transplantation the machine pressure should be maintained between 50 and 70 mmHg but the maximum pressure that is acceptable during deceased donor harvesting is not well-defined, although most researchers suggest that overflow of the irrigation of the pancreas tissue is very harmful to its future function [22].

In the adults, for prevention of micro- and macrovascular thrombosis, the standard dosage of heparin is 300 IU/kg and total volume of UW solution is 2–3 liter through the aortic cannula and 1 lit through the portal vein with a flow rate of 50–100 ml/kg/min for abdominal organ transplantation and another 1 liter for back-table preparation of the liver and at least 20 ml for irrigation of the bile ducts [23]. For lower viscosity solutions such as Celsior, HTK or IGL-1®, total volume of perfusate should increase to 6 liters [23] in order to achieve better irrigation of the total blood volume of the harvested organs. For pediatric donors the dosage of heparin is 500 IU/kg and total volume of perfusate should be around 50 ml/kg [23].

6. Cooling

Peritoneal cooling technique by slush ice is a safe and accepted old method for better organ function. It is a routine in all transplant units to use a perfusion temperature of 0–4°C for flushing all the organs but it is not widely proofed that the use of topical slush ice is really beneficial [24]. One author could prove that retroperitoneal slush ice may improve renal function [25] and another one showed improved islet cell recovery from pancreas grafts by using additional slush ice around the pancreas during the organ procurement [26]. There are so many reports in the literature about successful heart and lung transplantation after using topical ice. Transporting the organs in plastic bags filled with organ preservation solution and putting them into another ice –filled bag or cool box is the standard method of transferring organs between different transplant centers. Topical slush ice should be accepted as a routine until better prospective studies show another method but in all steps of organ procurement, preservation and transferring, it is extremely necessary to prevent organs' freezing with the use of good preservative solutions and prevention of direct contact of the ice to the tissues after retrieval.

7. Surgical procedure

7.1 General principles

Thomas Starzl and his team are the pioneer of multiple organ harvesting from the deceased donor and the technique that they described has minimal change till now after more than 3 decades [27]. All the procurement procedures have some steps in common:

i. Anesthesiologist management and use of muscle relaxant if needed

ii. Preparation and drape

iii. Long midline sternal and abdominal incision (with transverse extensions if needed)

iv. Primary evaluation of all the torso organs (with frozen section evaluations when indicated)

v. Control of the aorta for next step cannulation (abdominal; and thoracic if heart transplantation is planned)

vi. Control of supra-celiac and supra-iliac aorta for clamping (for better irrigation of abdominal organs with lower volume of preservative solutions)

vii. Warm dissection of all the important anatomic structures when indicated and the patient's hemodynamic is stable (for example portal vein, gastroduodenal artery, base of superior mesenteric artery and vein, renal arteries, veins and ureters, pulmonary artery and veins, bile duct, proximal and distal part of the duodenum, etc.)

viii. Preparation of the femoral, iliac vein or inferior vena cava (between the heart and liver, superior to renal veins, near its pelvic bifurcation) for evacuation of blood at the end of operation.

ix. Full heparinization (300/500 IU/kg)

x. Cannulation of aorta (abdominal; and thoracic if heart transplantation is planned); and portal vein if the patient is stable (through the superior mesenteric vein; or inferior mesenteric vein if short bowel transplantation is planned or cannulation of superior mesenteric vein is impossible or difficult)

xi. Clamping of supra-celiac, supra-iliac and thoracic aortic arc and beginning of irrigation and evacuation of blood through the previous large controlled veins and filling around of all organs with slush ice at the same time.

xii. Removal of the organs with this order: heart, lung, liver, pancreas, small bowel, kidneys, iliac and other large vessels, tissues with potential use as grafts (pericardium, bones, cartilages, tendons, skin, cornea, ...). This order may be changed according to planned transplantations and center expertise.

7.2 Starting the operation

Table 2 shows the checklist for essential pre-requisites of the donor characteristics before starting the operation. The surgical team should confirm that all the data in this checklist is ready and acceptable before starting the operation. Usually in most transplant units, the "liver team" is in charge of the whole operation and the operation is started by the most experienced and self- sufficient surgeon in this team by a long midline incision from jugular notch to symphysis pubis in the stable patient. In unstable patients all the steps of the operation may be omitted and replaced by femoral artery and vein cannulation for cold infusion of the preservative fluid and evacuation of the blood and after that all the dissections should be done after in situ cooling and aortic cross clamping below or above the diaphragm.

The time of the starting of the incision must be fully coordinated by all the other team members, coordinators and the in-hospital and out of hospital transport system to decrease the total ischemic time to the lowest possible time. It is better not to transfer the donor to other hospitals and in most countries, it is the procurement team that should go the donor hospital and they should have all the equipment, drugs, preservative solutions, organ bags, cool-boxes and surgical instruments that is essential with themselves. The leader of the team should finally check all the prerequisites of the organ donation operation including informed consent of donation,

Donor eligibility	
	Informed consent of donation by the next of keen
	Brain death confirmation by the authorities
Hemodynamic stability (ideal)	
	Central venous pressure 10–12 cmH_2O
	Systolic blood pressure maintenance >100 mmHg and mean arterial pressure >60 mmHg
	PaO_2 > 100 mmHg, SpO_2 > 95%, $PaCO_2$ between 35 and 40 mmHg and pH between 7.35 and 7.45
Urine output between 100 and 300 ml/hour	
No electrolyte imbalance	
	Na^+ < 160 and K^+ 3.5–4.5 meq/l
	Normal Ca^{2+}, Mg^{2++} and P
Negative viral tests	
	HBsAg, HCVAb, HIVAb, HTLV-1
No active infection	
No malignancy	
Normal organ specific function tests	
	Liver function tests, creatinine, histocompatibility tests results, echocardiography, ECG, angiography, bronchoscopy and Gram stains, chest imaging studies, insulin levels, etc.
Coordination with all the teams involved	
Readiness of all the recipients and their surgical team	
Availability of all surgical equipment needed	
Coordination with transport system	

Table 2.
Checklist for donor preparedness before starting the operation.

brain death confirmation (patient identity and certificate of death), important blood tests (especially the blood group and viral tests), previous history (especially history of untreated cancer and previous surgeries) and suitability of the donor just before the operation. Discussion of the steps of the operation with other teams will decrease potential injury to the retrievable organs.

A general physical exam is absolutely necessary because all palpable masses in the unexposed area such as breasts, genitalia, axillary and inguinal regions or any skin lesions which are suspicious for malignancies should be excised for pathologic examination.

Every surgeon has to use his or her maximum delicate surgical art to prevent any harm to any of the transplantable organs. For example, if the donor has previous midline sternotomy incision with potential adhesions of the heart, the thoracic incision should be delayed until all abdominal dissections are completed. Sternum may be incised by Gigli's saw or Stryker® sternal saw if available. After incision, complete hemostasis of all cutting surfaces is essential to prevent obscuring bleeding and suitable retractors such as large Finochietto retractors are placed for maximum exposure of the organs. All the organs should be explored for potential contraindications for donation such as congenital anomalies, malignancies or severe infective processes such as colon perforation or peritonitis.

7.3 Dissection of abdominal organs and large vessel cannulation

Every disturbing adhesion from previous surgeries should be released first to prevent jeopardizing the bowel wall. Superior mesenteric vein is dissected and controlled in the root of mesentery just to the right side of the Treitz ligament and the inferior mesenteric vein in the edge of this ligament. Cephalad retraction of the transverse mesocolon and caudal retraction of small bowel will better expose these two anatomic landmarks. After that, abdominal aorta and inferior vena cava (IVC) are fully exposed and controlled for cannulation by a complete right medial rotation of abdominal viscera from pelvic area till the infra-duodenal area superior to both renal veins. This step has to be done with caution to find all accessory renal arteries and prevent any inadvertent injury to lumbar arteries or veins which will result in uncontrollable or disturbing bleeding. If the distal aorta is not cannulable, the iliac arteries can be used instead. Inferior mesenteric artery (IMA) can be ligated and both ureters can be mobilized at this step but without any trauma to the tissues common between the ureters and genital veins.

Lesser sac is entered through the gastrohepatic ligament with caution not to injure potential left accessory hepatic artery. Left lateral segment of the liver is taken down from the diaphragm and supra-celiac aorta is exposed by blunt dissection of diaphragmatic crura and setting aside the abdominal esophagus and then controlled by an umbilical tape. If such dissections are impossible due to previous adhesions or any other reason, then thoracic aorta should be controlled in the left hemithorax just above the diaphragm and anterior to the lower thoracic vertebra.

At this stage, if "rapid flush technique" is chosen due to patient's instability, the operation is ended by full heparinization and aortic and portal cannulation, clamping the aorta and cutting the abdominal or infra-atrial IVC for blood evacuation along with the infusion of the preservative solution and covering all the viscera by slush ice.

If the patient is stable further dissections will be done. Bile duct is transected above the duodenum and flushed with 20 ml of cold normal saline. Cholecystectomy is performed. Gastroduodenal artery is explored in upper border of pancreas. If pancreas is suitable for transplantation, duodenum is prepared just next to the pylorus and after the pancreas uncinate process, posterior to transverse colon for transection at the end of operation and superior mesenteric artery is controlled just above the renal arteries root anterior to aorta. The cardiac team is now can come into the operation field.

7.3.1 *Tips and tricks*

In patients with history of heart surgery or median sternotomy, thoracic incision should be postponed till all the abdominal dissections and cannulation of the great vessels have been finished.

In patients with history of previous abdominal operations, incision should be started as far as possible from the site of previous incision to prevent bowel perforation.

In fatty donors, it is better to perform superior or inferior mesenteric vein dissections, because after full Kocherization and right medial visceral rotation, finding the mesenteric vein will be very difficult.

If during each step of the dissections, any vascular damage is encountered, it is better to repair it with fine sutures only if the location of the damage is easily found and repairable. In other cases, no attempt should be done, because it is time consuming and may cause further damage to critical organs.

During the cannulation of the aorta, the cannula should not be advanced above the celiac artery. Clamping the supra-celiac aorta at the end of the procedure will occlude the cannula and perfusion of the preservative solutions is stopped. All cannulas should have side holes for faster infusion of the solutions.

Unnecessary organ manipulations should be avoided to prevent vasoconstriction. In stable patients, some urologists insisted on postponing the rest of the operation when no urine is noted after ureteral transection.

7.4 Preparation of the heart

In stable donors, after the liver surgeon prepares all prerequisites in the abdomen the heart and/or lung team will welcome to the operation field. All thoracic lymphatic regions must be accurately inspected for signs of occult malignancies such as metastasis or lymphoma and if needed biopsy should be done and sent for frozen section pathologic examination. Thymus gland should be resected first and pericardium is opened longitudinally and fixed to the edges of transected sternum in both sides. Intraoperative cardiac evaluation includes inspection for: signs of previous pericarditis, hematoma or ecchymosis (resulted from previous cardiopulmonary resuscitation), any cardiac anomalies, dyskinesia, scars, contusions, calcification of ascending aorta and coronary arteries, size of the great vessels and heart chambers. At the same time, the inotrope dosage should be reduced by the anesthesiologist to ensure that cardiac contractility is good enough without need of the inotropes. If there is any sign of right heart overloud immediate diuresis by furosemide and reducing the central venous pressure by avoiding any intravenous infusion of crystalloids is mandatory. All the data should transfer immediately to the recipient team so they can make decision on starting the recipient operation.

The window between ascending aorta and pulmonary trunk is opened and controlled by an umbilical tape. Superior and inferior vena cava is encircled with caution not to harm the sinoatrial region or jeopardize the pulmonary veins. For cardioplegic injection at the end of preparation a cannula should be inserted and the arc of aorta should be prepared for clamping before the origin of the innominate artery.

7.5 Preparation of the lungs

Both pleural spaces should be opened at this stage. Lungs are inspected for bullae, contusions, atelectasis, pneumonia and occult tumors. Tracheal tube is disconnected and both lungs are deflated transiently and then inflated again by a pressure of 15–30 cmH_2O to better detect the pulmonary compliance (so called "collapse test") [28, 29]. Usually, most of the vascular dissections were done previous by the heart team including: separation of the pulmonary trunk and right pulmonary artery from posterior wall of the ascending aorta and superior vena cava, and opening the window between the lower right pulmonary vein and intrapericardial IVC (so called "oblique sinus"). The left innominate vein and artery is controlled by umbilical tape to expose the main trachea by retracting them toward the right and left, respectively. The azygous vein should be ligated at this stage to prevent rupture and bleeding. After inserting the cardioplegic cannula in the root of aorta and cannula should be inserted near the bifurcation of the pulmonary trunk for infusion of prostaglandin E1 and Perfadex for lung procurement at the end of all other organs' retrieval.

7.6 Common steps at the end of the procedure

When all dissections were done according to patient's stability and the retrievable organs prepared, great vessels' cannulation is done after full heparinization. The aorta is clamped at two levels: sub- or supra- diaphragmatic and at the end of ascending aorta. Blood evacuation is started by cutting the IVC just inferior to the right atrium or if dissections at this level is impossible, in the abdomen above the iliac vessels. Infusion of the cold preservatives (with cardioplegic effect if heart is being retrieved for transplantation) is started and supporting by the anesthesiologist is finished and the "definitive death" is announced. At the same time immersion of all the retrievable organ by slush ice should be accomplished. If lung procurement was programmed, infusion of Perfadex should be started at the same time and the pulmonary blood should be evacuated by cephalad retraction of the heart and incision of the left atrium between the two inferior pulmonary veins just below the Waterson's groove or "sulcus terminalis".

Infusion is continued till all the viscera are exsanguinated. Usually 2–3 lit of infusate through abdominal aorta, 1 lit through the portal vein, 1 lit for ascending aorta and 50 ml/kg of Perfadex is enough for complete blood evacuation. The superior mesenteric artery has to be ligated at this time for prevention of pancreas overperfusion which will severely affect graft function [30, 31]. If small intestinal retrieval is programmed, this step is forbidden, and portal perfusion should be omitted as well or performed through the IMV and only the aorta is perfused [30].

All the organs will be transferred after retrieval to an organ bag full of cold preservative and irrigated again if necessary. This bag should be packed and inserted to another bag filled with cold saline and again in the third bag full of slush ice and then in the cool box for transferring to the recipient ward or hospital. Sometimes especially when the transfer time is long or the donor is marginal the transplant team may decide to use cold or warm perfusion machines for better preservation of the organ.

7.7 Procurement of each organ

7.7.1 Heart and lung

Heart is easily retrieved by transecting the great vessels but this transection should be done step by step to prevent hematoma formation and injury to the vital parts especially the sinus node and pulmonary artery. When all the blood evacuated through the IVC incision, pericardium should be irrigated by cold saline at all steps to prevent warming. Cardioplegic cannula is removed. Aorta is cut just below the clamp, and SVC and IVC completely transected. The heart is gently pulled upward and inferior and superior pulmonary veins are divided one by one an at last the pulmonary trunk will be cut just at its bifurcation to remove the heart.

If the heart-lung complex is planned to be transplanted to one person, all these dissections should be avoided. The cardioplegia and pneumoplegia and prostaglandin E solutions is infused through the aortic and pulmonary artery catheters. Blood is evacuated from heart by incising the IVC and the returned blood from the lungs is evacuated through a small incision in left atrial appendages. Only the ascending aorta is transected before the innominate artery origin and the trachea is stapled after inflation of both lungs and removal of the endotracheal tube. The SVC is transected and origin of azygous vein is transligated and at last the heart -lung complex is procured by releasing their attachments to the mediastinum.

If transplantation of the lungs alone is planned, cardiac team should be left posterior wall of the left atrium intact in line with for pulmonary veins. After removing the heart, the posterior wall of left atrium and its surrounding pericardium is dissected from posterior mediastinum including the esophagus and descending and this avascular plate is continued till both lungs are released bilaterally. Small volume ventilation should be continued till all the dissections are completed and at the end and after complete inflation, the endotracheal tube is removed and trachea is stapled to extract both lungs outside the thoracic cavity.

7.7.2 En bloc retrieval of abdominal organs

The fasted way to retrieval of abdominal organs is en bloc resection. Sometimes the time is very important for the harvesting team for example when the organs will transfer to another city by a commercial flight. In some cases, all abdominal organs should be transplanted to one recipient, for example a recipient with cirrhosis due to complete portal and superior mesenteric vein thrombosis needs a simultaneous liver-small intestinal transplantation [32]. In such cases all abdominal organs have to be procured en bloc.

According to the organs being retrieved for multivisceral transplantation, there are several ways to do such procedure [30, 33]. After the heart and/or lung team retrieved their organs, the abdominal team can complete their operation. Amphotericin B, metronidazole and sometimes diluted povidone iodine is instilled into the duodenum by a nasoduodenal tube [31]. For better exposure and preventing of bowel content spillage, usually the stomach and colon should be resected and discarded first, by stapling the esophagogastric and gastroduodenal junction and also the ileocecal and colorectal junction and transecting their vasculature. Then the sub-diaphragmatic aorta which was previously controlled is transected. All diaphragmatic adhesions of the liver and spleen are released and the infra-atrial IVC is separated with a patch of pericardium and surrounding tissue around it. At last, all the organs including aorta, IVC, liver, pancreas, spleen and small intestine are swept up of posterior abdominal wall and lumbar vertebrae and muscles and the procurement is completed by transecting the ureters at pelvic rim and iliac vessels just before entering the femoral canal [3]. All the dissections in this step should be with extreme gentleness not to push or pull any of the vital structures.

7.7.3 Liver

In most centers liver and kidneys are the only organs used for transplantation especially when the donor has a high body mass index or marginal for any cause (unstable, diabetic, hypertensive, old age, etc.). For retrieval, these steps are necessary: transecting the infra-atrial IVC with a rim of pericardium and diaphragm, taking down the falciform, right and left triangular ligaments from the diaphragm, transecting the gastroduodenal (GD) and right gastric arteries and following the artery till the origin of the celiac artery by complete dissection of diaphragmatic crura.

If pancreas is not suitable for transplantation, dissection of the portal vein should be continued by transection of the pancreas neck anterior to SMV and swiping up the head of pancreas and duodenum to the right and the tail of pancreas to the left to expose the base of the SMV and SMA anterior to aorta. Then the origins of celiac and superior mesenteric arteries are separated from the aorta with a common Carrel patch. Replaced or accessory right and left hepatic arteries must not be jeopardized or pulled in any way and remained attached to their main large paternal vessel. Splenic vein and distal SMV SMA is transected at the level of uncinate process. IVC is transected above the renal veins' origin. Now after complete releasing of all inflow and outflow structures, the liver can be removed easily by final releasing it from the posterior wall and transferred to an organ bag and irrigated by another 1 lit of preservative solution without direct contact to ice.

If pancreas is transplantable all the dissections should be limited to upper border of the pancreas and portal vein and GD artery transected just above the duodenum and the SMV, SMA and splenic artery attachment to the pancreas be remained intact. Sometimes liver and pancreas will be removed in continuity and separated from each other in the time of back table preparation [30].

7.7.4 Small intestine

If gastrectomy and total colectomy were done previously with good hemostasis of the vessels, removal of the small intestine is relatively easy and straight forward. As I told before, at the start of the operation for exposure of the aorta and IVC, small intestine is gently wrapped in a lap-sponge and pull cephalad to detach all the mesentery in an avascular plain from ileum to the Treitz. At the end of operation and evacuation of all the blood by aortic and IMV irrigation, the small intestine only attached to the body superior mesenteric pedicle containing SMA and SMV. Duodenojejunal and ileojejunal junction was previously cut by staples and the whole graft can be removed only by cutting the SMA and SMV at this time. If small intestine is decided to transplant separately, it is necessary to remove it before liver and pancreas but if a multivisceral transplant is planned for the recipient, any dissection around the SMV and SMA at the root of mesentery is forbidden and IMV should be used for cannulation of the portal vein [30, 32, 33].

7.7.5 Pancreas

As I discussed previously, pancreas usually is procured along with the liver and separated from it in back table procedure. If the surgeon decided to retrieve each organ individually, then after removing the stomach by stapling of duodenum after pylorus, portal vein, GD and splenic arteries are cut at the upper border of pancreas. Another staple is used for transection of the duodenum between D2 and D3 area at the level of uncinate process, and the SMV and SMA and origin of mesentery is transected by another vascular staple. The IMV is ligated the lower border of pancreas is separated from left renal vein and the left kidney. The previously extended Kocherization is continued toward the left to separate the duodenum from the vertebra, aorta and posterior wall of the abdomen and at last the attachments of the spleen are released and procurement of the duodenum-pancreas-spleen is completed [30, 34].

7.7.6 Kidneys

Kidneys are the last organs that will be removed. They may be procured en-bloc in line with aorta and IVC when both of them are programmed to transplanted to one person (for example from a pediatric or marginal donor for an adult recipient, or when we encounter with a horseshoe kidney with multiple renal arteries and veins) or retrieved separately. For separation, IVC is transected transversely just above the renal vein origins and then incised longitudinally to explore for possible multiple renal veins. All renal veins should be separated with a common patch of IVC. Separation of renal veins should be done with caution not to injure the renal arteries which run posterior to veins especially accessory undefined renal arteries. Ureters (sometimes double or rarely multiple) are completely separated from the surrounding tissues and transected distally in the pelvic rim, but the window tissues between kidneys and ureters and also between the ureters and gonadal veins should remain intact to prevent ischemia and future contracture or anastomotic failure. Renal arteries are exposed by longitudinal incision of the aorta to find multiple branches from inside the aorta and retrieval with a common patch. Rarely an accessory branch may originate from the iliac arteries or the other side of the aorta. It is better not to jeopardize such branches but the kidney transplant team should be capable of back-table microvascular reconstruction of several arterial branches in such cases. Left adrenal vein is ligated and transected as well.

After complete separation of all arterial and venous branches, kidneys are retrieved by medial to lateral movement by the surgeon with extreme caution not to over-retract these branches and induce intimal rupture. Also rupture of renal capsule has to be prevented by using sharp dissections specially in older marginal donors. It is better to perform these dissections outside the perirenal fatty tissues to prevent such inadvertent injuries.

8. Machine perfusion

Full discussion about the machine perfusion is beyond the scope of this chapter. Ideally all the organs retrieved should be transplanted immediately or as soon as possible in the same center of the organ procurement. But this is impossible, irrational or illegal in many situations. The donor operation can be easily done in a small rural hospital without any transplant facilities in unstable patients. In such cases transferring the organ to other hospitals is the rule. Another such circumstances is, when histocompatibility (for example for kidney and pancreas), or duration of stay in the waiting list is an important matter for decision making, and transplantation in the same center in such cases is both irrational and illegal. In marginal donors and in cases of donation after cardiac death (DCD), it is very important for the transplant surgeon to predict functionality of the organs. In all such situation, machine perfusion is the best way to know the organ function and increase the time of organ viability before final *in vivo* reperfusion.

In contrast to static cold storage (SCD) which we discussed in all sections of this chapter, dynamic perfusion techniques use a perfusate for active perfusion of the organs *in situ* (*en vivo*) or ex situ (*ex vivo*) [35]. For example, normothermic regional perfusion (NRP) is an *en vivo* method for reconditioning organs for DCD by restoring oxygenated blood flow to the organs before procurement. For such purpose, we need a sophisticated Extracorporeal Machine Oxygenation (ECMO) technology, which is not available in most centers. In contrast to this technique, *ex vivo* machine perfusion is used after organ recovery specially for kidneys and liver. It may be used in a hypothermic (hypothermic machine perfusion or HMP) or normothermic (normothermic machine perfusion or NMP) milieu. For kidney grafts, it is shown that HMP reduced significantly delayed graft function both after DCD and donation after brain death in marginal donors [35]. NMP is an established method for confirming the functionality of marginal liver grafts by showing the function of the graft and preventing ischemic cholangiopathy and it is shown that this method reduced the discard rate by 50% [36]. The results are promising for pancreas and small intestine as well. Machine perfusion of the heart is an essential step in all cases of DCD and for lungs it is essential for uncontrolled DCD cases [37]. In my opinion, future of organ transplantation from marginal donors is in the hand of the engineers who invents better, cheaper and more efficient and reliable machines with simpler use by transplant surgeons, but at these days use of these techniques should be limited to high income countries with an extensive network of transplantation services all around their territories.

9. Conclusion

Multiorgan procurement from the same donor is the combination of the art of cooperation between several medical team with different expertise level. If any of the team member makes any mistake during such sophisticated procedure all other organs will be jeopardized and the life of many recipients will be in danger. It is the task of the team leader to manage such problems before they become irreversible, and this will be impossible without basic knowledge of all aspects of the other organ's retrieval by all other surgeons who is in charge of their organ.

Acknowledgements

This article is supported by Vice chancellor of research, Tabriz University of Medical Sciences, Tabriz, Iran. It is dedicated to my mentor great transplant surgeon Dr. Seyyed Ali Malekhosseini, the father of visceral transplant surgery in Iran.

Conflict of interest

There is no conflict of interest to declare.

Author details

Farzad Kakaei
Department of Surgery, Faculty of Medicine, Tabriz University of Medical Sciences, Tabriz, Iran

*Address all correspondence to: fkakaei@yahoo.com

IntechOpen

© 2020 The Author(s). Licensee IntechOpen. This chapter is distributed under the terms of the Creative Commons Attribution License (http://creativecommons.org/licenses/by/3.0), which permits unrestricted use, distribution, and reproduction in any medium, provided the original work is properly cited.

References

[1] Sayegh MH, Carpenter CB. Transplantation 50 years later--progress, challenges, and promises. *N Engl J Med*. 2004;351(26):2761-2766. doi:10.1056/NEJMon043418

[2] DeVita MA, Snyder JV, Grenvik A. History of organ donation by patients with cardiac death. *Kennedy Inst Ethics J*. 1993;3(2):113-129. doi:10.1353/ken.0.0147

[3] Frykholm R. Hjärndödsdebatten i Sverige. Aterblick, analys och nomenklaturförslag [Brain death debate in Sweden. Review, analysis and nomenclature proposals]. *Lakartidningen*. 1980;77(10):904-907.

[4] Tan SY, Linskey K. Christiaan Barnard (1922-2001): First heart transplant surgeon. *Singapore Med J*. 2019;60(10):495-496. doi:10.11622/smedj.2019127

[5] Sadler BL, Sadler AM Jr. Organ Transplantation and the Uniform Anatomical Gift Act: A Fifty-Year Perspective [published correction appears in Hastings Cent Rep. 2018 May;48(3):4]. *Hastings Cent Rep*. 2018;48(2):14-18. doi:10.1002/hast.834

[6] Shaw BW Jr, Rosenthal JT, Griffith BF, Haresty RL, Broznik B, Hakala T et al. Techniques for combined procurement of hearts and kidneys with satisfactory early function of renal allografts. *Surg Gynecol Obstet* 1983; 157: 261-264.

[7] Wright FH, Smith JL, Bowers VD, Corry RJ. Combined retrieval of liver and pancreas grafts: alternatives for organ procurement. Transplant Proc 1989; 21: 3522.

[8] Groth CG, Brent LB, Calne RY, et al. Historic landmarks in clinical transplantation: conclusions from the consensus conference at the University of California, Los Angeles. *World J Surg*. 2000;24(7):834-843. doi:10.1007/s002680010134

[9] Tzakis AG, Kato T, Nishida S, et al. The Miami experience with almost 100 multivisceral transplants. *Transplant Proc*. 2006;38(6):1681-1682. doi:10.1016/j.transproceed.2006.05.015

[10] Brockmann JG, Vaidya A, Reddy S, Friend PJ: Retrieval of abdominal organs for transplantation. *British Journal of Surgery* 2006; 93: 133-146. DOI: 10.1002/bjs.5228

[11] Kumar L. Brain death and care of the organ donor. *J Anaesthesiol Clin Pharmacol*. 2016;32(2):146-152. doi:10.4103/0970-9185.168266

[12] Mascia L, Pasero D, Slutsky AS, Arguis MJ, Berardino M, Grasso S, et al. Effect of a lung protective strategy for organ donors on eligibility and availability of lungs for transplantation: A randomized controlled trial. *JAMA*. 2010;304:2620-7. doi: 10.1001/jama.2010.1796

[13] Anwar ASMT, Lee JM. Medical Management of Brain-Dead Organ Donors. *Acute Crit Care*. 2019;34(1):14-29. doi:10.4266/acc.2019.00430

[14] Korte C, Garber JL, Descourouez JL, Richards KR, Hardinger K. Pharmacists' guide to the management of organ donors after brain death. *Am J Health Syst Pharm*. 2016;73(22):1829-1839. doi:10.2146/ajhp150956

[15] Granger P, Giolitto JP, Monod P, Descotes JL, Vialtel P, Rambeaud JJ *et al*. Multiorgan procurement (MPO). Who? How? What results?. *J Urol (Paris)* 1991; 97: 79-86.

[16] Wigmore SJ, Seeney FM, Pleass HC, Praseedom RK, Forsythe JL. Kidney damage during organ retrieval: data

from UK National Transplant Database. Kidney Advisory Group. *Lancet* 1999; 354: 1143-1146.

[17] Weissenbacher A, Vrakas G, Nasralla D, Ceresa CDL. The future of organ perfusion and re-conditioning. *Transpl Int*. 2019;32(6):586-597. doi:10.1111/tri.13441

[18] Jing L, Yao L, Zhao M, Peng LP, Liu M. Organ preservation: from the past to the future. *Acta Pharmacol Sin*. 2018;39(5):845-857. doi:10.1038/aps.2017.182

[19] Wahlberg JA, Southard JH, Belzer FO: Development of a cold storage solution for pancreas preservation. *Cryobiology. 1986 Dec; 23(6):477-82.*

[20] Latchana N, Peck JR, Whitson B, Black SM. Preservation solutions for cardiac and pulmonary donor grafts: a review of the current literature [published correction appears in J Thorac Dis. 2014 Sep;6(9):E207-8]. *J Thorac Dis*. 2014;6(8):1143-1149. doi: 10.3978/j.issn.2072-1439.2014.05.14

[21] Boteon YL, Laing RW, Schlegel A, et al. Combined Hypothermic and Normothermic Machine Perfusion Improves Functional Recovery of Extended Criteria Donor Livers. *Liver Transpl*. 2018;24(12):1699-1715. doi:10.1002/lt.25315

[22] Hamaoui K, Papalois V. Machine Perfusion and the Pancreas: Will It Increase the Donor Pool? *Curr Diab Rep*. 2019;19(8):56. Published 2019 Jul 10. doi:10.1007/s11892-019-1165-y

[23] Keutgen XM, Petrowsky H. Procurement for visceral organ transplantation: where to cannulate and how to perfuse? *Current Opinion in Organ Transplantation*. 2014 Apr;19(2):92-99. DOI: 10.1097/mot.0000000000000066.

[24] Ostróżka-Cieślik A, Dolińska B, Ryszka F. Tips for optimizing organ preservation solutions. *Acta Biochim Pol*. 2018;65(1):9-15. doi:10.18388/abp.2017_2312

[25] Salazar-Bañuelos A, Monroy-CuadrosM,Henriquez-CooperH. Retro-peritoneal cooling for kidney preservation from multi-organ cadaver donors. *Am J Surg*. 2018;215(5):802-803. doi: 10.1016/j.amjsurg.2017.12.015

[26] Lakey JR, Kneteman NM, Rajotte RV, Wu DC, Bigam D, Shapiro AM. Effect of core pancreas temperature during cadaveric procurement on human islet isolation and functional viability. *Transplantation*. 2002;73(7):1106-1110. doi:10.1097/00007890-200204150-00016

[27] Starzl TE, Miller C, Broznick B, Makowka L. An improved technique for multiple organ harvesting. *Surg Gynecol Obstet*. 1987;165(4):343-348.

[28] Pasque MK. Standardizing thoracic organ procurement for transplantation. *J Thorac Cardiovasc Surg*. 2010;139(1):13-17. doi:10.1016/j.jtcvs.2009.09.015

[29] Nguyen DC, Loor G, Carrott P, Shafii A. Review of donor and recipient surgical procedures in lung transplantation. *J Thorac Dis*. 2019;11(Suppl 14):S1810-S1816. doi:10.21037/jtd.2019.06.31

[30] Abu-Elmagd K, Fung J, Bueno J, Martin D, Madariaga JR, Mazariegos G, Bond G, Molmenti E, Corry RJ, Starzl TE, Reyes J: Logistics and Technique for Procurement of Intestinal, Pancreatic, and Hepatic Grafts From the Same Donor Ann Surg. 2000 Nov; 232(5): 680-687. doi: 10.1097/00000658-200011000-00010

[31] Ricordi C, Mazzeferro V, Casavilla A, Scotti C, Pinna SA, Tzakis PA, Starzl TE: Pancreas procurement from multiorgan donors

for islet trasplantation. *Diabetes Nutr Metab*. 1992;5(S1):39-41.

[32] Busuttil RW, Farmer DG, Shaked A, et al. Successful combined liver and small intestine transplantation for short-gut syndrome and liver failure. *West J Med*. 1993;158(2):184-188.

[33] Bharadwaj S, Tandon P, Gohel TD, et al. Current status of intestinal and multivisceral transplantation. *Gastroenterol Rep (Oxf)*. 2017;5(1):20-28. doi:10.1093/gastro/gow045

[34] Samoylova ML, Borle D, Ravindra KV. Pancreas Transplantation: Indications, Techniques, and Outcomes. *Surg Clin North Am*. 2019;99(1):87-101. doi:10.1016/j.suc.2018.09.007

[35] Weissenbacher A, Vrakas G, Nasralla D, Ceresa CDL. The future of organ perfusion and re-conditioning. *Transpl Int*. 2019; 32:586-597. doi:10.1111/tri.13441

[36] Nasralla, D., Coussios, C.C., Mergental, H. *et al.* A randomized trial of normothermic preservation in liver transplantation. *Nature.* 2019; 557: 50-56. doi:10.1038/s41586-018-0047-9

[37] Van Raemdonck D, Rega F, Rex S, Neyrinck A. Machine perfusion of thoracic organs. *J Thorac Dis*. 2018; 10(Suppl 8): S910-S923. doi:10.21037/jtd.2018.02.85

Chapter 4

Thoracic Organ Procurement during Multi-Organ Retrieval

Suresh Keshavamurthy, Vipin Dulam, Eros Leotta, Mohammed A. Kashem and Yoshiya Toyoda

Abstract

Procurement of thoracic organs can be divided into two major categories- donation after brain death (DBD) or donation after circulatory determination of death (DCDD). In this section we will focus primarily on DBD, which is the commoner of these two or at times referred to as standard procurement. DCDD is a relatively new and promising field that has helped ameliorate donor shortage, aided by the latest advances in medical technology. However, DBD continues to be the major avenue of organ donation. There are several different combinations of thoracic procurement surgeries: heart, double lung, single lung/ 2-single lungs, heart-lung en bloc for transplantation, Double Lung procurement for Bronchial arterial revascularization, Heart and Lung procurement in DCDD donors with the OCS, NRP or Lungs for EVLP.

Keywords: thoracic organ procurement, multi-organ harvest, DCD

1. Introduction

We believe that procurement is 50% of the transplant operation and deserves due emphasis. Often times it is assigned to a junior member of the team and consequently impacts the outcome due to the learning curve involved. We have put together our experience to serve as a road-map to help improve the art and science of procuring thoracic organs for transplantation [1].

In the first section of this chapter we will focus primarily on DBD, which is the commoner of these two or at times referred to as 'standard procurement.' We will expound on Heart, Lung/s and combined Heart-Lung procurement.

2. Donation after brain death

2.1 DBD: heart only procurement

First, we will focus on an isolated heart procurement. This is with the understanding that it is the sole organ being procured from the chest.

The surgeons must first familiarize themselves with the donor's vital signs, ECG, ECHO, angiogram, labs and any other form of imaging that's available in order to assess the hemodynamic stability and anatomy of the donor to avoid surprises. Perhaps even more importantly, donor blood type and match information must be confirmed. These are (but not limited to) the donor's MHC status, antibody checks, and ABO blood type compatibility. Other donor information such as Hepatitis B, Hepatitis C, and HIV status should also be double checked in the donor chart on site. Discrepancies should be conveyed to the rest of the transplant team at the recipient site immediately. The suitability of the organ with respect to size match in terms of a predicted heart mass ratio should be confirmed. At the site, a copy of the consent for donation and the donor's brain death status as per the specific state's legislated criteria are to be obtained for the procurement surgery teams records. Finally, confirm that the donor had no other changes in status since the procurement team's original debrief and arrival at the site. Specifically, the surgeon must look out for worsening lab values, such as changes in the lactate levels, and any increase in pressor requirements. The usage of Thyroxine (T4) as part of the donor recruitment process is also recommended [2].

The procurement team's next step should be to assess if there is appropriate arterial and venous access for the donor. At times one sees that the donor only has a femoral arterial access line. This leaves the patient without any blood pressure monitoring when the abdominal team ligates the aorta during their cannulation. Because of this, the anesthesia team can get alarmed and give boluses of pressor medications, which in turn can have a deleterious effect on the heart. Therefore, we recommend upper limb invasive pressure monitoring system such as a radial artery line or brachial arterial access.

The sternum is opened via a median sternotomy in a standard fashion limiting blood loss and securing hemostasis. It is our practice to measure intracardiac pressures from the Right Atrium, Left Atrium and Pulmonary Arteries from the donor heart to get an accurate estimate of the patient's hemodynamics. These parameters are immediately communicated to the implanting surgeon. These measures give the team a snapshot of the cardiac function of the donor's heart.

The heart surgeon will have to share the IVC with the liver surgeon. This can be a point of contention regarding the length of IVC to be taken by the cardiac surgeon versus the length taken by the liver transplant team. An ambitious cardiac surgeon might divide the IVC at the level of the diaphragm with traction on the heart to the extent where the IVC retracts below the diaphragm and leaves but a stump for the liver transplant team. Hence, it is prudent to discuss with the liver surgeon beforehand as to where to transect the IVC. Staying above the diaphragmatic reflection has been the standard practice. Avoiding traction while harvesting is important, though one often sees the liver team retracting the liver down!

The procurement surgeon should pay special attention to the venting that is done to decompress the donor heart. With multiple teams sitting in the fray, this aspect of the surgery is often ignored at the patient's peril. The techniques to vent the heart are either through the LA appendage, the interatrial groove, the posterior left atrial wall or directly amputating the pulmonary veins [3]. In this scenario, where we are discussing heart only procurement, it is useful to vent through the pulmonary veins (the pulmonary vein orifices can be connected in the back table). However, if other thoracic transplant teams (like the lung team) are involved then they will be perfusing the lungs with 4–6 liters of Perfadex *(PERFADEX® Plus is an extracellular, low potassium, dextran-based electrolyte preservation solution for rapid cooling, perfusion and cold static storage of donor lungs – pre-supplemented with calcium ions and THAM*; Perfadex® Goteborg, Sweden solution). Our experience shows that it is best to vent through the left atrial appendage. Venting through the interatrial groove can also be done (must be dissected out before the cross-clamp application) but it comes with a major hazard- the heart may go into atrial fibrillation and cause hemodynamic compromise. Venting primarily through the posterior left atrial wall is also an option.

For this, the surgeon first picks up the heart to access that portion of the left atrium but once the opening is made and the heart is let down back into its position in the chest cavity, it is not predictable if the hole will stay open to adequately vent the heart. Furthermore, lifting the heart during cardioplegia administration might cause aortic sufficiency. The pulmonary veins can be amputated at their origins and we can divide the pulmonary artery as high as we need to in order retain the bifurcation. It is also wise to divide the SVC high up above the azygos vein to give the implanting surgeon additional SVC length.

These are special situations in which it is important to know the anatomy of the recipient and to discuss with the implanting surgeon specific requirements.

3. Adult congenital heart disease recipients

Recipients of Adult congenital heart disease needing heart transplantation for advanced heart failure have generally undergone multiple open-heart procedures in the past. Therefore, they might need additional donor tissue to reconstruct the recipient anatomy.

In those recipients with an anomalous left superior vena cava (LSVC), the implanting surgeon will need extra length of the SVC and also need to harvest the innominate vein to allow for restoration of continuity of the LSVC in the recipient [4]. On the other hand, in the donors with an LSVC one must be extra conscious of the donor heart vasculature. There have been noted cases where the coronary sinus drains into the LSVC instead of the RA [5]. Ligating the LSVC without ascertaining drainage to the RA could prove to be disastrous for the recipient because after implantation and circulation restoration, the heart has no drainage avenue and hence may become edematous and lead to primary graft dysfunction. Any additional systemic/pulmonary venous drainage anomalies are also important to note on both the recipient and donor.

For certain circumstances, such as a recipient with complex congenital heart disease who may require reconstruction of the pulmonary arteries, additional tissue may need to be procured either in continuity with the donor heart or separately, such as the descending thoracic aorta or innominate vein. If possible, the PA bifurcation along with the RPA and LPA should be procured if the lungs are not being placed [6].

If possible for these subset of patients it is important to procure a long length of the donor aorta till the arch, the PA with the bifurcation and extra lengths of RPA and LPA, donor carotid artery, descending thoracic aorta, donor pericardium, etc. to aid reconstruction and repair in the recipient.

4. LVAD explants/redo chest

Since these patients have an outflow graft placed on the ascending aorta. The procurement surgeon must harvest the ascending aorta as distal as possible past the three arch branches in the donor. This gives the implanting surgeon enough length and flexibility to decide where to do the aortic anastomosis.

5. Heterotopic heart transplant

This chapter mainly focuses on orthotopic heart transplantation (the standard explant of the old diseased heart, and implant of a new donor heart into the chest cavity). However, there is another form of heart transplant which has been performed since the 1970's called heterotopic heart transplantation [7]. While this is rare, there are few select indications for this procedure, and we wanted to include this for completion.

An extra length of aorta is required, and the pulmonary veins must be transected close to their origin to give the recipient surgeon enough room to operate with. The procuring surgeon must also take as much of the SVC/IVC as possible. The Pulmonary Artery will need to be augmented with a graft material in the recipient because the implanting surgeon will connect the pulmonary artery of the new heart to the pulmonary artery of the recipient's native heart. Therefore, it becomes extra important to take as much of the pre-bifurcation PA as possible.

6. Final steps

After explantation of the heart, the surgeon should check for a patent foramen ovale (PFO); if one does exist, then a PFO closure using a 4–0 prolene suture should be performed as quickly as possible before putting the heart in the cooler. Inspect the pulmonary artery and aorta, mitral valve, tricuspid valve for any anatomical abnormalities/clots/vegetations/iatrogenic damage. At this point, inform the recipient surgeon if there is any injury. If there is, then donor pericardium can be packed to repair these injuries in the recipient OR.

Some teams prefer to leave the cardioplegia cannula attached to the donor aorta. In these centers the cardioplegia cannula can be placed lower down on the aorta. However, if the cannula is removed and the suture tied to mark the point of cannulation, the cannulation site can be higher up and the same can be excised/trimmed prior to implantation.

Pack the heart in the preservative solution and ensure it is completely immersed in it. The first bag should not contain any ice, while the second and third bags do contain ice. There are special containers that maintain uniform cooling of the heart (Paragonix SherpaPak™) in 4 degrees centigrade [8]. These containers help to optimize donor heart transport by maintaining uniform cooling and perhaps extend the donor warm ischemia time.

6.1 DBD- procurement of heart and lung for separate centers

In this section we want to discuss procurement of both the lungs and the heart as separate organs from the same donor but for different recipients. (Note: the procurement surgeon however might still be from the same center) In this scenario, the heart is being taken for transplant, while simultaneously, the lungs are being procured either as double lung, single lung, or two single lungs. This implies that both the heart surgeon and lung surgeon (unless one surgeon is taking both for two separate patients in the same center) will be present.

Assuming that each of the two lungs are being taken by different centers, and the heart is being taken by another center, up to three different surgeons could be present for procurement of the thoracic organs. It requires the utmost cooperation and communication with each other to be able to successfully execute such a multi-organ procedure.

We recommend the heart surgeon start first and inspect the heart. The sternotomy is performed in the midline once all teams are present, signed in and the basic checks are conducted. Hemostasis is achieved using ample amounts of bone wax. The pericardium should be split down the middle. Three pericardial stay sutures should be put on either side of the pericardial opening and tag them to hemostats. Based on our practice we recommend that the pericardial stay sutures not be hitched up to the drapes at this point. The reason for this is it causes tension on the pericardium, and when the lung surgeon is trying to inspect and recruit the lungs with a Valsalva maneuver it squeezes the heart to cause hemodynamic compromise [9].

Once the heart is appropriately visualized, the heart surgeon should check the quality of the heart by palpating the coronary arteries to assess for atherosclerosis, visually confirm the heart's contractility, and by checking the right atrium, the right ventricle, the pulmonary artery and the aorta. It is also important to check if there are any palpable thrills or any anomalies in the systemic venous drainage or pulmonary venous drainage. Our practice is to measure the intracardiac pressures; the PA, RA, and LA and communicate them with the implanting surgeon for cross check. It is important to avoid opening the pleura. This is when the lung surgeon steps into the limelight.

Once the lung surgeon approaches the table, the pleura should be opened widely. We recommend opening the pleura bluntly rather than using the diathermy. We have seen many instances where opening the pleura by a diathermy causes an air leak because it accidentally punctures the lung surface. These air leaks are difficult, notorious, and persistent. After one part of the pleura is opened bluntly, then the surgeon can insert one finger behind the pleura but above the lung tissue. The surgeon can now safely use a bovie with the finger protecting the lung in order to divide the rest of the pleura in standard fashion. At this stage inspect the lungs and recruit and atelectatic areas. The lung surgeon is now ready for Valsalva. After communicating this with the anesthesiologist, the lung surgeon reaches for the lower lobe, lifts it up and gives Valsalva at 30 cmH2O pressure [9]. It is important to refer here to the earlier point about leaving the pericardial stay sutures unhitched. If they had been hitched and the lung surgeons performed the Valsalva, the heart will get compressed between the hitched-up pericardium and the lung/s. This would cause a precipitous drop in blood pressure. Therefore, leave the pericardial stay sutures unhitched, and incise the pleura widely, so that the heart has more room to move. Once the lung surgeon has ascertained the quality of the lung by checking its compliance, and inspecting any abnormalities such as masses or contusions, then the stay sutures can be hitched up on either side. Depending on institution protocol, pulmonary vein blood gases are taken from the right upper, right lower, left upper and left lower pulmonary veins making sure the ventilator settings are on fiO2 of 100% and PEEP of 5.

The procurement then resumes in standard fashion. First the surgeon dissects the aorta and the pulmonary artery, then uses an umbilical tape to loop the aorta, while separating the svc from the pulmonary artery. Then the surgeon loops the SVC and ligates the azygos vein (this step is optional). The azygos vein is fragile and can be easily injured precipitating brisk bleeding which is difficult to manage. We prefer not to dissect the IVC or interatrial groove before heparin is given so that we avoid hemodynamic compromise and rhythm disturbances such as atrial fibrillation. Therefore, it is prudent to always have internal defibrillation paddles on the sterile table opened and ready to use during procurement. Standard dose of heparin is then given- 30,000 units (adjust according to patient weight). Then the cardioplegia stitch is taken, and the aorta is cannulated. We suggest a dual lumen cardioplegia cannula and transduce the pressure line to monitor the aortic root pressure of the patient. This helps us by telling us the cardioplegia perfusion pressure (ideal is 60–80 mmHg) [10].

Once the heart surgeon cannulates the aorta, the lung surgeon places the purse string on the PA. At this point the surgeons must decide where to divide the Pulmonary artery. On the one hand, one would want to keep an adequate length for the heart surgeon, so it is important to not cut it too short On the other hand, one would want to leave the bifurcation of the PA intact for the lung surgeon. Therefore, we usually use the right pulmonary arteries a guide and place the purse string suture at that level. Once the purse string suture is placed, we suggest using a right angle canula and directing the bevel of the cannula towards the pulmonary valve. The reason for this is to avoid improper perfusion of the pulmonary arterial flush. Often, novice procurement surgeons do everything correctly except turn the bevel of the cannula towards the left PA. This results in preferential flow into the left lung with minimal flow into the right lung, which causes mal perfusion with improper protection of the right lung. If using a different type of cannula, it is still important to ensure adequate distribution of the pulmoplegia.

Once all the teams are ready, the heart surgeon cross clamps the aorta and the lung surgeon administer the prostaglandin. The injection site should be as close to the purse string suture on the PA as possible to avoid additional puncture to that artery. This is when all the teams should be extremely alert because the prostaglandin causes the BP to drop. Then, the SVC is snared, and the left atrial appendage is divided by placing a Satinsky clamp on it and the tip is amputated. It is important not to put traction on the LAA while placing the clamp to avoid injury to the base of the appendage or Left Circiumflex artery. For this reason, some surgeons are averse to the idea of placing a clamp on the LAA [11].

However, if they are venting through the interatrial groove, then that that should be done first before dividing the IVC. The next step is to divide the anterior wall of the IVC. Wait for about 3–4 beats after this is done to. Be patient as the heart empties, and cross clamp the flaccid heart's aorta as distally as possible towards the arch vessels and start the infusion of the cardioplegia solution. Please note that it is not until the heart is noticed to be fully arrested that the lung team can start the Perfadex solution - be aware to not start them simultaneously. Meanwhile, the surgeon should be constantly observing the heart- feeling the left ventricle to make sure its soft and feeling the aorta to make sure it is firm.

When the Pulmoplegia is being perfused into the PA, note that one should see the efflux through the Left atrial appendage. Keep monitoring the color of the lungs to look for uniform blanching indicating even distribution of the flush solution whilst continuing to ventilate the lungs and simultaneously dropping the FIO2 to 50%. Avoid manipulating the heart during this process. If the LV distends for any reason, stop the cardioplegia and the pulmoplegia, release the cross clamp on the aorta and gently decompress the heart. and then reapply the cross clamp and resume cardioplegia, and pulmoplegia. If the distension continues, open the LA appendage more. If that still does not work, use the interatrial groove to vent. Usually around 4–6 liters of the perfadex solution is given but it varies per hospital protocol.

Keep the cardioplegia running if the perfadex is running. This makes sure the perfadex does not enter the coronaries and wash out the cardioplegia. If the cardioplegia is done before the pulmoplegia, then an aortotomy should be made while the clamp is still there, and a yonkaeur sucker should be inserted into the aorta to suction out and avoid any perfadex solution going into the heart. Once all the flush is done for both the heart and lung, the pulmonary artery cannula is removed, and the prolene suture is cut away. The IVC is then completely divided, taking care to avoid any injury to the right inferior pulmonary vein.

The next step is optimal division of the left atrium. Our recommended approach is to gently retract the heart up while we incise the posterior LA wall and proceed using a Metzenbaum scissors to enlarge the incision leaving an adequate cuff of LA for the lungs at least a 1 cm rim. On the right side, stop the dissection as you reach the IVC. At this point, we recommend the heart be retracted to the left. With the flaccid heart and bloodless field, it should be easier to dissect out the interatrial groove. and leave at least a one-centimeter cuff for the lung implant [12].

Finally, we can transect the aorta as high as possible depending on how much aorta is needed. For the PA extend the incision from where it has been cannulated. Visualize the carina of the PA. Make sure you can see the opening of the right PA. Divide the PA in such as fashion that the bifurcation remains with the lung block. Do not use too much traction while dividing the PA because that can cause distortion. Make sure that the original cut is perpendicular as to leave adequate PA for the heart team. Now that all the divisions are done, release the snare on the SVC, divide the SVC, the azygos vein and anything else holding the heart behind as it is gently lifted out.

The lungs are then harvested in standard fashion. It is always helpful to have the nasogastric tube so that one can feel the esophagus. The arch vessels and innominate artery are divided, at which point the trachea is exposed and looped. The trachea is then stapled at 60% tidal volume. The lungs are then taken to the back table and given 250 cc's of retrograde flush through each pulmonary vein [13]. There are different ways of effectively conducting the retrograde flush. Some do it in situ in the chest, while others take the lung bloc to the back table. We prefer taking it to the back table and use 250 cc's of perfadex per vein so in total about a liter of retrograde flush (amongst all four veins).

One technique is a foley catheter with an inflated bulb at the tip; inserted into each vein sequentially as the flush is administered. The caveat with this is that one may inadvertently injure the pulmonary vein ostium (which is delicate) by excessively distending it. The other technique, personal communication from Dr. Hassan Nemeh at Henry Ford Health System, is to use a retrograde cardioplegia catheter which has a self- inflating balloon, so it is much more elegant and less traumatic [14]. The only problem with this is it is not part of the standard kit, so the procurement surgeons must remember to bring it with them. Yet another technique that can be used is to utilize the rubber tubing that comes on the end of tubing. Insert the tube into the pulmonary vein and then pinch the vein to provide a tight seal. Whichever technique may be used, note that it is important to have the perfadex solution only 30 cm above the table and run it by gravity; avoid delivering it at excessive pressure which can lead to pulmonary edema!

When the retrograde flush is being perfused be sure to inspect the pulmonary artery for any clots. It is not uncommon to see tiny emboli. If, however large clots are seen, it is important to alert the implanting surgeon who might either choose to abandon or repeat a retrograde flush at the implanting center. Some teams are utilizing EVLP in such situations. After completion of the retrograde flush look inside the PA to assess if there are any clots remaining.

6.2 Heart Lung en Bloc

'Heart-Lung en Bloc' transplantation surgery has become less frequent over the years (Lund LH, Khush KK, Cherikh WS, Goldfarb S, Kucheryavaya AY, Levvey BJ, et al. The Registry of the International Society for Heart and Lung Transplantation: Thirty-fourth Adult Heart Transplantation Report-2017; Focus Theme: Allograft ischemic time. J Heart Lung Transplant. 2017;36(10):1037-46). However, there are still select indications for it, and one should be aware of how it is performed. The procurement surgeon performs the assessments for both heart and double lungs (as discussed in the earlier section) and oversees physiological and anatomical assessments both for the heart and lungs. The heart assessment is made in standard fashion- the coronaries are palpated, the aorta is inspected, the right atrium and pulmonary artery are assessed, and any palpable thrills are ruled out. Look thoroughly for contusions and note any evidence of trauma. Injuries which could impact implantation should be thoroughly discussed with the rest of the team. Once the assessment is complete and the heart is deemed good for transplant, we proceed to assess the lungs in standard fashion. Our assessment includes bronchoscopy, ventilatory mechanics, compliance and gentle recruitment followed by selective pulmonary vein blood gasses done on a vent setting of 100% fiO_2 and PEEP of 5 cmH_2O.

Administer heparin to do the donor as soon as all the teams are ready. The aorta is then canulated, and the PA cannulation follows shortly after (as described earlier, the bevel should be turned towards the pulmonary valve). It is important that the pulmoplegia (Perfadex) be kept no higher than 30 cm off the table thereby letting it run by gravity.

Once all the teams are ready for cross clamp, prostaglandin is injected into the PA. The heart is vented through the left atrial appendage. A major notable difference from the double lung procurement is that there is no retrograde flush; only an anterograde flush is done. The SVC (superior vena cava) is snared above the level of the azygos vein; the azygos vein would have been ligated earlier. The IVC is partially transected at a point of agreement with the liver team.

It is prudent to patiently wait for the heart to empty, and then cross clamp the ascending aorta right below the innominate artery. We suggest not clamping the aorta when the heart is still ejecting. After this, start the cardioplegia infusion, while also measuring the aortic root pressure and wait for the heart to arrest prior to starting pulmoplegia (Griffith BP, Magliato KE. Heart-lung transplantation. Operative Techniques in Thoracic and Cardiovascular Surgery. 1999;4(2):124-41). As soon as the flush is started, we cover the heart, lungs, and entire pleural cavity with ice slush. All the while be aware that the heart is not distending, that the aortic root is firm, the LV is soft and of course that the LA appendage is adequately draining. Look at lung surfaces to see that they're evenly blanched.

Request the Anesthesia team to decrease the FiO_2 to 50% and ventilate the lungs for proper distribution of pulmoplegia to all the lobes. Again, it is important to keep an eye on the LV to make sure it is not distending. Avoid lifting the heart so as not to cause aortic insufficiency! Ensure there is a backup cardioplegia bag in case of a hypertrophied LV. Avoid pulmoplegia going into the coronaries! Either keep the root distended with additional cardioplegia or transect the aorta and place a yonkaeur sucker till the pulmoplegia is done.

Once the cardioplegia and the pulmoplegia are done, the pulmoplegia cannula is removed and the purse-string suture is secured. Similarly, the cardioplegia cannula is removed and the suture secured depending upon institution preference. We then complete the inferior vena cava (IVC) transection and then transect the ascending aorta as high as possible. We then divide the inferior pulmonary ligaments on both sides and complete the division of the posterior pericardium. It is important to keep the nasogastric tube so that we can palpate and tell where the esophagus is to not contaminate the mediastinum. Be sure to dissect anterior to the esophagus and go up to the level of the azygos vein and then divide the azygos vein.

Now for the final steps. Loop the trachea as high as possible. After a few recruitment breaths, the endotracheal tube is withdrawn, and trachea is stapled at 60% of the tidal volume. Then we divide the SVC as high as possible near junction of innominate vein, taking care to avoid retaining a piece of central line while transecting the SVC. Now we have IVC, SVC, Aorta and trachea all divided. Important not to have more than 60% of the tidal volume to avoid barotrauma. The heart lung bloc is delivered onto back table. Quick inspection is made for iatrogenic injuries. The heart lung bloc is then packed in the heart solution. Have adequate solution enough to immerse the entire bloc. The inner bag contains only the preservative solution, while the second and third bag have ice slush. The heart-lung is then labeled accordingly and packed in the cooler for transportation. It is important to communicate to the implanting surgeon the conduct of the harvest and update him about any iatrogenic injuries and need for repairing the left atrial appendage venting site.

7. Donation after circulatory death

7.1 DCDD- lung only procurement surgery (heart not placed for transplant)

Once an offer for a DCDD lung is received the surgeon and the pulmonologist will process the offer just like a standard one. More specifically, the blood gasses, the X-Ray, the CT scan (if not available, request one), the ventilatory timeline, and the bronchoscopy findings (not always done) should all be analyzed. The nature of the donor death should also be scrutinized very closely- such as drowning or hanging [15].

The key in assessing a DCDD lung offer in comparison to a standard DBD offer is that the target PaO2 is 350 mmHg as a rule out. In our clinical practice, we currently do not venture to inspect a DCD lung unless the p/f ratio is adequate [16]. Using 350 mmHg is a good starting point especially in those centers where DCD volume is not very high. There are few centers who place all DCDD lungs on EVLP and have different set of guidelines. For a DBD offer we would venture to inspect the lung even with a PaO2 of 300 mmHg or lower. The reason for this discrepancy is that in a standard DBD we have the ability to recruit the lung, assess it, check the blood gases and decide in the operating room if the lung is suitable for transplantation. In DCD- what we have is what we get- so we must ascertain the lung status before we head over to the center, which explains why we have more stringent cut-off: to make sure that the lung is acceptable radiologically (CT scan preferred) and physiologically. Bronchoscopy is often done after withdrawal of care (most of the time it is for flushing) and it is done in a rush [6].

In conclusion we must be very careful with the pre-operative assessment in a DCD lung. There are certain centers, especially Toronto, where all the DCD lungs are put on EVLP. Hence it does not matter what the PaO2 ratio is [17]. They then evaluate these lungs while on EVLP, but not all centers have that luxury yet. Before a DCD Lung transplant procurement is initiated at the recipient center, the following questions should be asked in a checklist format:

1. Where is life support being withdrawn? ICU/OR (**Figure 1**)

2. Is there adequate central vein access

3. Will the patient be extubated? Is it acceptable to disconnect the ventilator and leave the tube-suspected difficult intubation?

4. Will they leave the NG/OG on suction?

5. What is the institution policy after withdrawal-certification; when can the team start-quiescent period?

6. Will they permit bronch prior to withdrawal?

7. How much heparin is being given? Is it at least 30,000 units. If not then plan to add 50,000 units into the first bag of perfadex.

8. When is the heparin being administered? Ideally it should be at least 3–5 minutes prior to withdrawal of life support.

9. Are there at least 2 wide bore functioning suctions available and adequate amount of soft slush available?

10. Does the center have a functioning sternal saw and chest spreader- preferably a transplant spreader (one with spikes)

For the actual withdrawal of life support, it is preferable to have 2 surgeons on the lung procurement team. Withdrawal is initiated by removal of the endotracheal tube, however in some cases when there is extensive airway edema due to potential difficulty in securing airway, the ventilator is disconnected instead after discussion with the anesthesiology team.

Of note, it is important to have the nasogastric tube (NG) maintained on continuous suction during the withdrawal of life sustaining therapy. This action prevents aspiration of gastric contents and facilitates dissection near the esophagus [18]. It is also important to communicate the importance of the NG to the anesthesia team before extubating. The surgical team is then scrubbed and ready in the adjacent

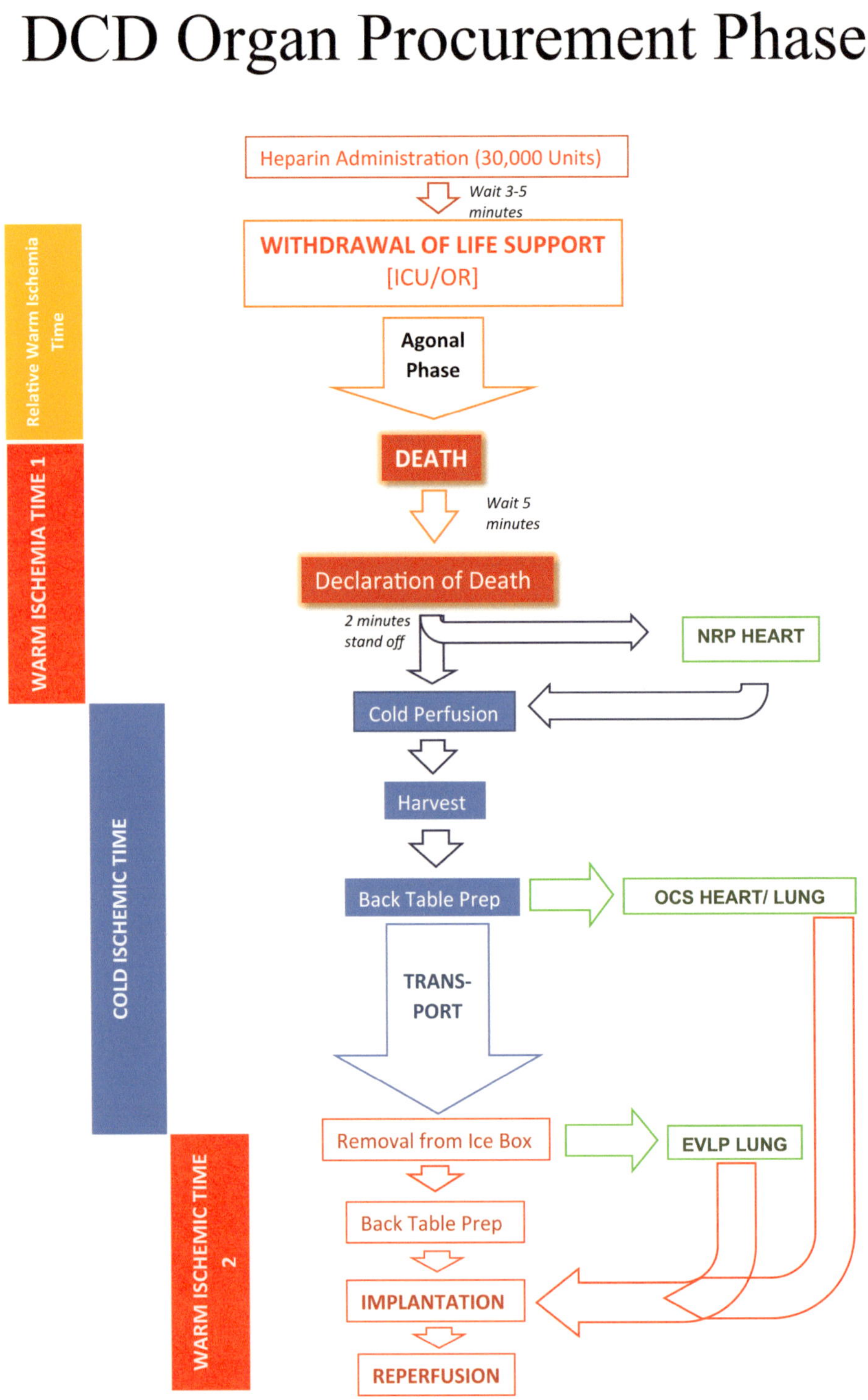

Figure 1.
DCD-Donation after circulatory death, ICU-Intensive care unit, OR-Operating Room, NRP-Normothermic Regional Perfusion, OCS-organ Care system, EVLP-Ex-vivo lung perfusion.

operating room or sterile corridor. The patient is prepped and draped in sterile fashion with a hand being left out for the family if they are coming into the operating room to pay their last respects. A sterile sleeve is made available for the stethoscope usage to auscultate and declare death. The flush solution is prepared by injecting prostaglandin into the first bag of Perfadex [19]. The lines are then passed off the sterile field, hung on the IV pole, and then accessed. Alternatively, the flush bags can be kept in the ice box at the side of the table after being reconstituted and spiked.

Death is declared as per local hospital protocol. The patient is then re-intubated. Median sternotomy is performed, and the pericardium is opened by pick up technique with forceps and scissors. (Please note that there is no bovie used during a DCD procurement!) The IVC is then vented by partial transection in a location previously discussed with the liver procurement team.

At this juncture the Liver team is frantically trying to clamp the descending thoracic aorta in the chest if they do not have access below the diaphragm. The thoracic team can help by quickly opening the left pleura, releasing the inferior pulmonary ligament, mobilizing the lung, then looping the descending thoracic aorta bluntly and helping to place the cross clamp so that they can start perfusing the abdominal organs. We can then focus on perfusing the lungs.

8. Techniques of pulmonary artery flush

1. Often times we have found in our experience that it is easy to use a straight, stiff cannula (a femoral arterial cannula) especially when there is a single surgeon or there is insufficient help. Using a #15 blade a small nick is made in the RVOT just enough to permit the cannula entry and the cannula is introduced into the PA after advancing across the pulmonary valve. This effectively delivers equitable antegrade PA flush and obviates the need for a purse string and effectively holds the cannula in place.

2. When qualified help is available, a 4–0 Prolene purse string suture is placed on the main pulmonary artery just below the bifurcation/more towards the RVOT. Using a #11 balde an arteriotomy is performed. This is then gently dilated with a tonsil/Schnitz and a right angled/straight cannula is inserted. If angled, then ensure the bevel is pointing towards the pulmonary valve. The cannula is connected to the Perfadex flush solution. The ascending aorta is cross clamped, the left atrial appendage is amputated and 60–70 ml/kg of Perfadex is then infused in antegrade fashion. Both pleural cavities are widely opened bluntly with fingers and the chest cavity packed with soft ice. After the patient is re-intubated by the Anesthesiology team/second surgeon, the lungs are then ventilated with tidal volume of 6-8 cc/kg and fiO2 of 50%. The second surgeon then proceeds with bronchoscopy while the first surgeon continues with the flush. If only one surgeon is available, then take this time to re-intubate. Proceed to then ventilate and bronch while the flush runs and the chest is adequately packed in ice.

Following instillation of the Perfadex solution, the cannula is removed. The lungs are then recruited with Valsalva maneuver at 30 cm H2O and both lungs are sequentially examined in standard fashion. The heart is then excised in standard fashion. In certain instances, there is consent for homograft valves and sufficient care needs to be exercised while excising the heart to preserve the valves [20].

Next, dissection begins first by dividing the inferior pulmonary ligament (bilateral) and the posterior pericardium. The main and right pulmonary artery are dissected away from the aorta. Bilaterally, the inferior pericardium is then divided at the level of the esophagus. Then the posterior pericardium is divided in a horizontal fashion just above the esophagus to the level of the pulmonary veins. The aortic arch is then transected. The superior aspect of the arch is then exposed and divided as distal as possible along the arch vessels so that a portion of the wall of the arch and descending aorta are left as a cuff to prevent dividing the ligamentum arteriosum.

Attention is then turned to the trachea which is isolated just above the carina with blunt dissection. A TA-30 stapler is passed around the trachea 3 rings above the carina [21]. The lungs are inflated to 60% tidal volume-to avoid baro-trauma (especially if the lungs are being flown back to the recipient institution), and the endotracheal tube is withdrawn. The stapler is used to divide the trachea. The lung bloc is removed from the donor after division of any remaining attachments.

The lung bloc is taken to the back table. Retrograde flush is performed at 250–500 cc/vein x4. If lot of clots/thrombi are seen exiting the PA during retro flush one can take a call regarding quality (small clots are not uncommon).

The double lung bloc is then examined for compliance, color, any areas of inadequate perfusion, atelectasis etc. (refer to DBD procurement of lungs section). Once the procurement surgeon is satisfied that the lungs are suitable for transplantation the recipient surgeon is called, and if accepted the lungs are then split on the back table and packed in standard fashion. The main PA is divided at the insertion site of the pulmonary artery cannula. The atrial cuff is then created approximately 1 cm from insertion of the pulmonary veins into the left atrium. The atrium is then divided in the midline with scissors. The left mainstem bronchus is divided with a TA-30 stapler near the hilum. An additional liter of cold Perfadex solution is instilled bilaterally via the pulmonary veins with a balloon catheter. The lungs are packed first in a bag containing Perfadex, followed by 2 bags containing ice cold saline slurry. The organs are subsequently transported to their respective transplant centers.

8.1 If only 1 surgeon performing procurement

If only 1 surgeon is available on the procurement team, the steps occur as described until flush occurs with the Perfadex solution. The chest is then packed with ice and ventilation continues. The lung procurement surgeon will scrub out. The surgeon will then along with the anesthesia team intubate the patient, perform bronchoscopy, and initiate ventilation. The surgeon will then scrub back in and continue to harvest in the previously described fashion.

8.2 DCD heart only placed for transplantation (OCS)

The process of DCD heart only procurement with Organ care system (OCS) is a relatively new technology, which will be discussed in this section. For this procedure, it is very important to ensure that two surgeons are present as part of the procurement team. The reason for this will become more relevant as the discussion of the technique ensues. After the patient's hemodynamic status, drips, lactates, troponins, echo, and other vital parameters have been checked out the procurement team proceeds to the donor center and there the traditional checklist is followed. These include (but are not limited to) the blood groups and that the UNOS IDs being checked. At that point, the procuring team and the local organ procurement organization (OPO for short) will familiarize themselves with the local institutional/hospital protocol. The donor team will park the Transmedics-organ care system (OCS) in one of the corners of the operating room, plug in the power, ready the equipment and will ensure that every object, instrument, and machine is given a green signal for the procedure. The patient is prepped and draped in sterile fashion and all lines are passed off. The cardioplegia is spiked and ready to be infused at short notice. We make sure that there is a functioning sternal saw, a sternal retractor and the appropriate aortic cross-clamp. Lastly, we ensure there are 2 working and connected suctions.

About 3–5 minutes before withdrawal of care, 30,000 units of heparin are given intravenously into a central vein in the donor. The donor procurement team will then scrub in and be ready while they wait in the sterile corridor. Upon withdrawal of life support the OPO coordinator will communicate the hemodynamic status of the donor (which is the arterial blood pressure and pulse oximeter) to the team at every 5 minutes intervals. For the DCD heart while there is no set or accepted timing. From what we have seen generally, 18–23 minutes of waiting time is acceptable. Beyond this time, the heart team deems that there has been a prolonged ischemia phase. Hence, the wait time is limited to 23 minutes. In totality, the mandatory 5 minutes after cessation of electrical activity (before the patient was pronounced) and the 1–2 minutes time before the team is permitted to start brings the total time to around 30 minutes. This is the time interval beyond which the cardiac team would walk. The liver team generally waits for 30 minutes while the lung team has a more permissive waiting period of up to 60 minutes.

Then the surgical team comes in, with all their instruments already on a side table right next to the operating table. Using a knife, an incision is made all the way down to the bone. The next item is the sternal retraction. Once the sternotomy is done, the retractor is placed, and the pericardium is opened in the midline using forceps and a scissor. The heart is exposed at that point and the right atrium is cannulated with a 32 French venous cannula and this is then connected to that blood collecting bag which was handed off to the perfusion team member. He/she will then collect 1100 cc of blood at least (800–1100 cc of blood from the donor will be collected).

In the meantime, a purse-string on the aorta and a cardioplegia needle is placed in the ascending aorta. Once we have completed blood collection, the aorta is cross-clamped, and we then infuse cardioplegia in standard fashion. We give 2 L of cardioplegia into the aortic root and we then packed the chest with ice. The IVC is vented and from that point on the tip of the left atrial appendage is also amputated. From that point on the procurement proceeds in standard fashion. The IVC is incised at the point where the liver team and the cardiac team agree to. Once the cardioplegia is completed, the pulmonary veins are anterior rated, the IVC transaction is completed, the pulmonary arteries are divided beyond the bifurcation of the IO at the level of the aortic arch. The SVC is divided as high as possible above the level of the azygos vein and the heart is finally explanted and is then taken onto the back table. There, instrumentation is done to place the heart on the OCS machine. We will encourage readers look for that part of the information as it is beyond the purview of this chapter.

9. Bronchial artery revascularization

Bronchial Artery Revascularization has been done to alleviate the Achilles heel of lung transplantation which bronchial healing. This has been an area of intense focus especially since the early issues that lung transplantation had with tracheal dehiscence and bronchial dehiscence. However, it is very labor intensive and has not taken off as a major standard of practice yet. There are a few proponents of this technique who have shown excellent results [22]. One of these groups is the Cleveland Clinic, championed by Prof. Gosta Pettersson who has worked on it for a long time since his days in Denmark. He has trained several surgeons in the Cleveland Clinic with this approach [23].

As one is aware, the lung has dual blood supply. One is from the bronchial arteries and one is from the pulmonary arteries. The major idea of the BAR procedure is to procure the lungs as we normally do, but to also retain the bronchial arteries from their origins in the aorta. In order to achieve this, the lungs are removed en bloc with the trachea intact like they are in a standard procedure, except this time the thoracic esophagus and descending aorta accompany them as well. This way, the RICBA and left bronchial arteries are included.

After IV heparin administration, the donor aorta is cross clamped and cold lung perfusate is administered via the PA. Normally we flush the lungs with 4–6 L of perfadex. 4 Liters are used for antegrade perfusion and then 1 Liter perfadex for retrograde perfusion on the back table. One liter of perfedex must be infused into the descending aorta. A cross clamp should be put on the aortic arch to keep the solution from escaping. This ensures perfusion of the bronchial arteries which come off the descending thoracic aorta. The NG tube is pulled back (but not all the way, because it is still important to keep it in the esophagus) before stapling the esophagus off- this is to ensure the NG tube is not stapled inside the esophagus. Then one must go around to the aorta and transect it at the level of the diaphragm. To prevent spillage the esophagus must be also be stapled off as high as possible at the neck. Keep in mind that one must try to minimize the dissection around the trachea. The trachea is also stapled off as high as possible [22].

Finally, the double lung bloc and its accompanying tissue is excised from the donor while moving cranially. Be sure to include the paraspinal tissue as well to minimize any possibility of injury to the bronchial arteries. The PA is divided near its bifurcation, and sufficient left atrial cuff is harvested in standard fashion.

After arrival in the recipient operating room, the esophagus is separated on the back table. After the esophagus is removed, the descending aorta is opened vertically in the midline and the bronchial arteries identified. The surgeon must locate the RICBA and the left bronchial artery. The use of a coronary probe can help in this matter. The RICBA is identified in the right. On the right, once the RICBA is identified, clips are applied to its intercostal branch. The left bronchial artery (or arteries) is/are identified with probing if needed. On either side, a single bronchial artery of reasonable size is usually sufficient for complete revascularization. However, if a convincing bronchial artery is not identified or if an important bronchial artery is damaged, BAR should be aborted and standard bilateral sequential LTx should be performed [22].

Author details

Suresh Keshavamurthy[1*], Vipin Dulam[2], Eros Leotta[3], Mohammed A. Kashem[3] and Yoshiya Toyoda[3]

1 Division of Cardiothoracic Surgery, Department of Surgery, University of Kentucky College of Medicine, Lexington, KY, USA

2 Lewis Katz School of Medicine, Philadelphia, PA, USA

3 Division of Cardiovascular Surgery, Department of Surgery, Temple University Hospital, Philadelphia, PA, USA

*Address all correspondence to: suresh.keshavamurthy@uky.edu

IntechOpen

© 2021 The Author(s). Licensee IntechOpen. This chapter is distributed under the terms of the Creative Commons Attribution License (http://creativecommons.org/licenses/by/3.0), which permits unrestricted use, distribution, and reproduction in any medium, provided the original work is properly cited.

References

[1] Mooney, J.j., Medlin H, Mohabir PK et al. "Donation After Circulatory Determination of Death Donor Characteristics and Lung Donor Utilization Within the United States." *The Journal of Heart and Lung Transplantation*, vol. 34, no. 4, 2015, doi:10.1016/j.healun.2015.01.785.

[2] Salim A, Vassiliu P, Velmahos GC, et al. The Role of Thyroid Hormone Administration in Potential Organ Donors. *Arch Surg.* 2001;136 (12):1377-1380. doi:10.1001/archsurg.136.12.1377

[3] Sudhir Sundaresan, MD, Gregory D. Trachiotis, MD, Motoi Aoe, MD, G. Alexander Patterson, MD, and Joel D. Cooper, Donor Lung Procurement: Assessment and Operative Technique MD Division of Cardiothoracic Surgery, Department of Surgery, Washington University School of Medicine, Barnes Hospital, St. Louis, Missouri

[4] Tyrak KW, Holda J, Holda MK, Koziej M, Piatek K, Klimek-Piotrowska W. Persistent left superior vena cava. *Cardiovasc J Afr*. 2017;28(3):e1-e4. Published 2017 May 23. doi:10.5830/CVJA-2016-084

[5] Kurtoglu E, Cakin O, Akcay S, Akturk E, Korkmaz H. Persistent Left Superior Vena Cava Draining into the Coronary Sinus: A Case Report. *Cardiol Res*. 2011;2(5):249-252. doi:10.4021/cr85w

[6] Copeland, H., Hayanga, J.W.A., Neyrinck, A., Macdonald, P., Dellgren, G., 2020. Donor heart and lung procurement: A consensus statement. The Journal of Heart and Lung Transplantation.. doi:10.1016/j.healun.2020.03.020

[7] Erwan Flécher, Olivier Fouquet, Vito Giovanni Ruggieri, Céline Chabanne, Bernard Lelong, Alain Leguerrier, Heterotopic heart transplantation: where do we stand?, *European Journal of Cardio-Thoracic Surgery*, Volume 44, Issue 2, August 2013, Pages 201-206, https://doi.org/10.1093/ejcts/ezt136

[8] Michel S.G., LaMuraglia G.M., Madariaga M., Anderson L.M. (2015). Innovative cold storage of donor organs using the Paragonix Sherpa Pak ™ devices. *Heart, Lung and Vessels, 7*, 246-255.

[9] Kumar C.M., Van Zundert A.A.J. Intraoperative Valsalva maneuver: a narrative review. *Can J Anesth/J Can Anesth* **65,** 578-585 (2018). https://doi.org/10.1007/s12630-018-1074-6

[10] Lopes JB, Santos CCMD Júnior. Coronary Perfusion Pressure during Antegrade Cardioplegia in On-Pump CABG Patients. *Braz J Cardiovasc Surg*. 2017;32(3):171-176. doi:10.21470/1678-9741-2017-0035

[11] Katona A, Temesvári A, Szatmári A, Nemes A, Forster T, Fontos G. Left circumflex coronary artery occlusion due to a left atrial appendage closure device. *Postepy Kardiol Interwencyjnej*. 2015;11(1):69-70. doi:10.5114/pwki.2015.49192

[12] McAlpine WA. Heart and Coronary Arteries. Berlin/Heidelberg: Springer-Verlag; 1975:58-59.

[13] Hayama M, Date H, Oto T, Aoe M, Andou A, Shimizu N. Improved lung function by means of retrograde flush in canine lung transplantation with non-heart-beating donors. J Thorac Cardiovasc Surg. 2003 Apr;125(4):901-6. doi: 10.1067/mtc.2003.296. PMID: 12698154.

[14] Vigneswaran, W. (Ed.), Garrity, E. (Ed.), Odell, J. (Ed.). (2016). Lung Transplantation. Boca Raton: CRC Press, https://doi.org/10.1201/b19234

[15] Rao V, Dhanani S, MacLean J, et al. Effect of organ donation after circulatory determination of death on number of organ transplants from donors with neurologic determination of death. *CMAJ*. 2017;189(38):E1206-E1211. doi:10.1503/cmaj.161043

[16] Keshavamurthy S, Murthy SC, Pettersson GB, Mason DP. Lungs from donation after cardiac death for transplantation. Eur J Cardiothorac Surg. 2013 Jul;44(1):189. doi: 10.1093/ejcts/ezs696. Epub 2013 Jan 15. PMID: 23321432.

[17] Machuca TN, Cypel M. Ex vivo lung perfusion. *J Thorac Dis*. 2014;6(8):1054-1062. doi:10.3978/j.issn.2072-1439.2014.07.

[18] Metheny NA, Clouse RE, Chang YH, Stewart BJ, Oliver DA, Kollef MH. Tracheobronchial aspiration of gastric contents in critically ill tube-fed patients: frequency, outcomes, and risk factors. *Crit Care Med*. 2006;34(4):1007-1015. doi:10.1097/01.CCM.0000206106.65220.59

[19] Salizzoni S, Toyoda Y. Effects of Prostaglandin E1 and Nitroglycerin on Lung Preservation In: Principles of Pulmonary Protection in Heart Surgery. Springer London; 2010:81-89. Doi: 10.1007/978-1-84996-308-4_9

[20] Herreros JM, Mastrobuoni S, Ubilla M, Rábago G, Lorente Ruiz M, Rifón J, Hernández M. Trasplante de homoinjertos valvulares cardiacos y vasculares [Cardiac and vascular homograft valves transplant]. An Sist Sanit Navar. 2006;29 Suppl 2:153-61. Spanish. PMID: 16998523.

[21] Chekan E, Whelan RL. Surgical stapling device-tissue interactions: what surgeons need to know to improve patient outcomes. *Med Devices (Auckl)*. 2014;7:305-318. Published 2014 Sep 12. doi:10.2147/MDER.S67338

[22] Yun JJ, Unai S, Pettersson G. Lung transplant with bronchial arterial revascularization: review of surgical technique and clinical outcomes. *J Thorac Dis*. 2019;11(Suppl 14):S1821-S1828. doi:10.21037/jtd.2019.09.09

[23] Pettersson GB, Karam K, Thuita L, Johnston DR, McCurry KR, Kapadia SR, Budev MM, Avery RK, Mason DP, Murthy SC, Blackstone EH. Comparative study of bronchial artery revascularization in lung transplantation. J Thorac Cardiovasc Surg. 2013 Oct;146(4):894-900.e3. doi: 10.1016/j.jtcvs.2013.04.030. Epub 2013 Jun 29. PMID: 23820173.

Section 3

Immunological Aspects of Organ Transplantation

Chapter 5

Pathology of Intestinal Transplantation: Rejection and a Case of Tolerance

Tatsuaki Tsuruyama

Abstract

Small bowel transplants are less common than other organ transplants. Histological criteria for rejection of the transplanted small intestine were proposed at the 8th International Symposium on Small Intestinal Transplantation 2003-2004. The Banff Conference on Transplant Disease Pathology, an international conference on the rejection of small bowel transplants, was held in 2019, and unifying diagnostic criteria were discussed (https://banfffoundation.org/pittsburgh-2019/). These histological criteria are expected to be standardized in the near future. This review outlines new findings such as apoptosis and apoptotic-body phagocytic findings in the lamina propria and behavior of natural killer T (NKT) cells, in addition to previously known crypt Fas-related apoptosis in acute cellular rejection. Furthermore, we review the case of a recipient who has shown no rejection for 5 years after transplantation. In the transplanted small intestine of this patient, the lymphocytes were replaced by those of another male patient.

Keywords: intestinal transplantation, histology, rejection, natural killer T cells, apoptosis, tolerance

1. Introduction

1.1 Current status of small bowel transplantation

Small bowel transplantation (SBT) is one of the standard treatments for patients who are unable to consume a regular diet and have complications from the irreversible requirement of parenteral nutrition [1]. Hirschsprung's disease [2, 3] and Crohn's disease [4] patients are two examples. Recent effective immunosuppressive drugs, well-controlled postoperative care, and advances in diagnostic techniques have significantly improved the outcome of SBT [5]. Immunosuppressants such as mycophenolate mofetil, tacrolimus, and steroids, are routinely used for long-term management after transplantation [6, 7].

Acute cellular rejection (ACR) is a major cause of impaired colonization by the transplanted small intestine, and it frequently accompanies chronic and irreversible changes such as ulcers and lamina propria fibrosis. ACR has remained a risk factor that impedes functional recovery of the intestinal graft [1, 8, 9]. On the other hand, pathologists frequently encounter various pathologies of the intestinal allograft [10–12]. For example, mechanical failure of the graft due to operation during

IntechOpen

surgery may occur during the early phase after transplantation. Cytomegalovirus (CMV) enteritis and Epstein–Barr virus -related enteritis are severe side effects and post-transplantation lymphoproliferative disorders/diseases [13–15]. It is often difficult to make a differential diagnosis of the ACR findings. However, histologic diagnosis is critical for the selection of immunosuppressants and their respective doses. Tacrolimus, cyclosporin, and steroids are commonly prescribed in the early stages of rejection [16]. If an excessive dose is administered, the occurrences of CMV enteritis and EBV enteritis become inevitable.

Among the various histological features, crypt epithelial cell apoptosis has been evaluated as a highly reproducible finding. However, other histological findings have been proposed at different institutions. We have also previously suggested other findings as indicators of ACR [17–19].

2. Diagnostic criteria for ACR

2.1 Crypt apoptosis

Crypt apoptosis is considered a unique feature of ACR in SBT. The crypt is an architectural element that is located at the base of the villous epithelium and serves as the source of mucosal cells. Paneth cells, stem cells, and reserve stem cells are included in the crypt. Enterocytes are differentiated from reserve stem cells in the crypt and migrate to the tips of villi through the transit amplifying zone [20]. The kinetics of differentiation and loss of enterocytes contribute to the maintenance of quick renewal for mucosal homeostasis. The supply of enterocytes becomes interrupted by apoptosis in the crypt, and the shortening of villi becomes unavoidable. When ulceration occurs, the lesion is susceptible to infectious enteritis such as CMV- and EBV-related enteritis, for a significant period of time [21, 22].

Pathologically, the diagnosis of small bowel transplant rejection is based on the appearance of 6 or more apoptotic lesions per ten crypts [3, 4] (**Table 1**). The detection of crypt apoptosis is commonly used because of its high reproducibility. Nevertheless, discussions about the number of lesions per crypt were held at the Banff Conference 2019. In the case we experienced, if more than six apoptotic cells were detected in the crypts, subsequent ulceration is inevitable, and infection from the ulcer site might occur. Therefore, we considered that immunosuppressants should be administered when apoptotic cells were observed in the crypt [18].

Previous apoptosis findings have shown that the cells are eosinophilic with an intensely stained nucleus [17, 18] (**Figure 1**). Cells with lobulated nuclei, such as neutrophils and apoptotic cells, can be confused morphologically; therefore, careful observation is necessary. Terminal deoxynucleotidyl transferase dUTP nick end labeling (TUNEL) staining is one method to avoid this confusion. This staining procedure involves an enzyme-mediated reaction. First, the fragmented DNA is labeled with biotin containing terminal deoxynucleotidyl transferase. The labeled DNA then reacts with streptavidin for staining. Both labels with 3,3′-diaminobenzidine (DAB) and fluorescein isothiocyanate (FITC) are available for visualization of the apoptotic body [18].

As apoptosis progresses, fragmented cell debris (apoptotic bodies) are observed in or around the crypt. Increasing the dose of the immunosuppressive drug suppresses the progression of apoptosis. Therefore, quick detection of apoptosis is critical for effective immunosuppression therapy [18, 19].

The factors that cause such apoptotic responses in the crypt and lamina propria are poorly understood. It is possible that cytotoxic T lymphocytes (CTLs) can directly

Histologic grade			
Indeterminate	Crypt apoptosis and related findings	Lymphocytic apoptosis in the lamina propria [18]	
	Up to 6 apoptotic bodies per 10 crypts	None	
Mild	>6 apoptotic bodies per 10 crypts Confluent apoptosis	Isloated apoptotic bodies in the lamina propria	Phagocytosis of apoptotic bodies by macrophages [18]
Moderate	Increased inflammation, epithelial injury	A few apoptotic body cluster in the lamina propria	Aggregation of macrophages [18]
Severe/exfoliative	Mucosal ulceration	Apoptotic bodies aggregate in the lamina propria	Granuloma consisting of macrophages

Table 1.
Histological criteria for ACR of the intestinal allograft [10]. The findings under the lymphocyte and macrophage categories refer to our previous study [18].

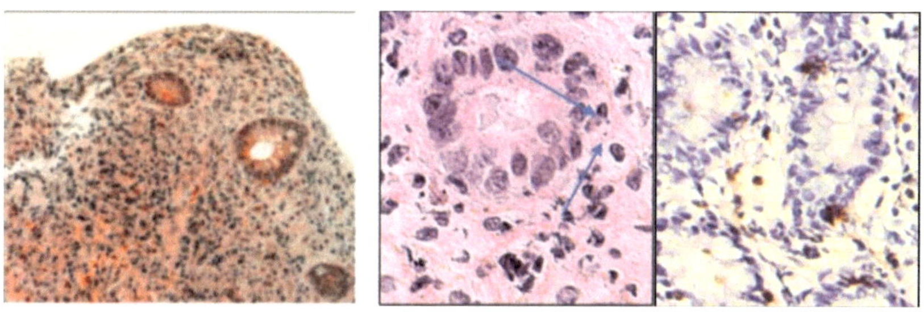

Figure 1.
Histology of ACR of the intestinal allograft. The onset of ACR. Eosinophil infiltrates are observed in the ulcerated mucosa (left, 100×). Apoptotic bodies are observed in the crypt (indicated by arrows, middle, 200×; right, 100×, TUNEL-stained with 3,3'-diaminobenzidine).

attack the crypt of the graft. However, it is not always histologically evident that CTLs directly infiltrate near the crypt and remain near this area. There is also a noteworthy research report suggesting that CD8-positive CTLs are not always involved in ACR [23]. At the basic research level, rejection of the apoptosis-inducing factors perforin and granzyme B released from CTLs has been reported [24]. Therefore, the destruction of the mucosal immune system by local increases in complement and inflammatory cytokines is thought to be the cause of apoptosis.

2.2 Immunohistochemical monitoring

In addition to the crypt apoptosis, apoptotic lymphocytes are identified by systematic immunostaining of lymphocyte surface antigens: T cell surface antigens CD3, CD4, and CD8; B cell surface antigens CD20 and CD79a; natural killer cell surface antigen CD56; and activated lymphocytes Fas and its ligand (FasL) [25]. FasL, also known as CD95L, is a surface antigen of activated cytotoxic T cells and NK cells are observed at the onset of rejection [18] (**Figure 2**, upper panels).

Apoptotic bodies are also been observed in the lamina propria and Peyer's patch (PP) distant from the crypt, and the macrophages that phagocytose them often aggregate to present granuloma-like findings. Notably, these bodies are stained with

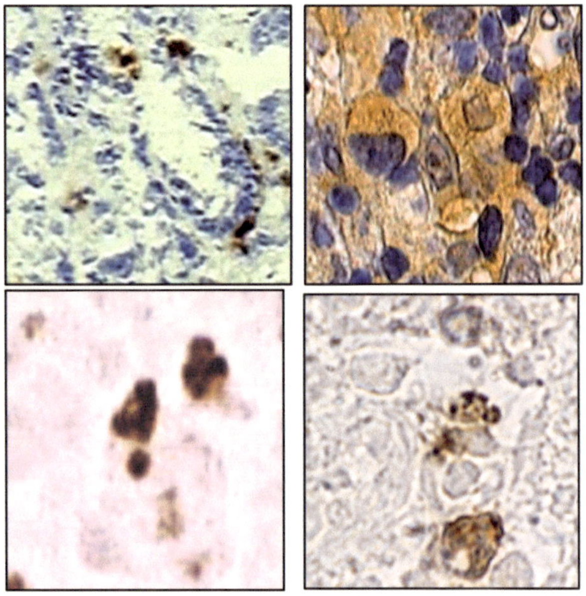

Figure 2.
FasL immunostaining of the intestinal allograft. FasL-positive lymphocytes in the lamina propria (upper left, 200×) and Peyer's patch (upper right, 400×) are shown. FasL-stained apoptotic bodies (lower left, 400×). Apoptotic TCRVα24 stained cells (lower right, 400×). TCRVα24 and FasL were visualized with DAB (3,3'-diaminobenzidine).

FasL and Fas, suggesting that the apoptosis relates to the FasL-Fas interactive reaction (**Figure 2**, lower panels). This result was first reported in our previous study [18].

3. Endoscopic examination and Peyer's patch response

Endoscopically, elevation of the small intestinal mucosa may be recognized and biopsied when clinical rejection is suspected. Since this elevation is observed in patients who are not receiving oral nutrition, the change may not be the result of irritation from the lumen of the small intestine and more likely due to the reaction of the Peyer's patches (PPs) to a load of patient cells on the graft mucosal immune system. In our cases, the biopsied Peyer's patches were injured at the onset of ACR (**Figures 3A** and **B**). Therefore, PP is one of the targets of ACR or other types of rejection (**Figure 3C**). Notably, B cells increased in number in the disintegrated PPs (**Figure 3**). As described later, IL-5 was increased in the intestinal allograft [17], which may promote the transient B cell growth in PP.

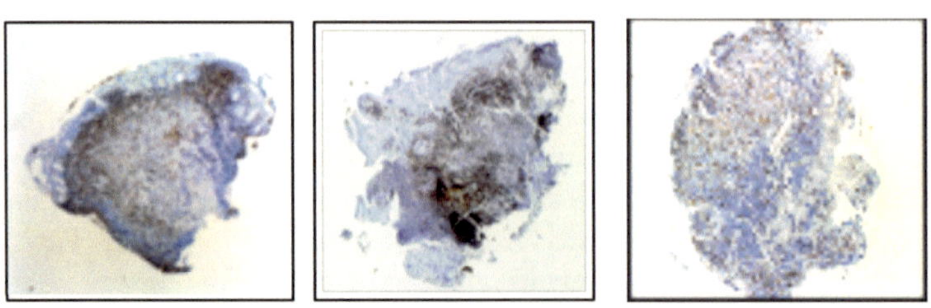

Figure 3.
Histology of a PP in an intestinal allograft. (A, B) A hyperplastic Peyer's patch stained with CD79a antibody before ACR (A) and at the onset of ACR (B). (C) CD8 staining of PP after 42 h at the onset of rejection. Many CD8+ CTLs infiltrate in PP. CD79 and CD8 were visualized by DAB. The photo magnitude is 100×.

4. Cases at Kyoto University Hospital

Here we review cases of SBT at Kyoto University Hospital [17, 18, 21, 22]. SBT was performed owing to intestinal malrotation and Hirschsprung's disease-related effects (**Figure 4**).

Jejunal or ileal grafts were monitored histologically. When fever, increased intestinal juice, abdominal pain, or C-reactive protein (CRP) elevation in peripheral blood (>0.5 mg/10^{-1} L) was observed, an endoscopic examination was performed. In particular, for the first 1 to 2 weeks after surgery, the examination was performed every other day, and a histological examination was also performed. Once the condition of the patient became stable, a histological examination was performed approximately once a week, and the state of the intestinal graft was monitored continuously for up to 2 months in the hospital. The patient received immunosuppressive therapy in combination with tacrolimus (trough concentration: 20 ng/mL) and methylprednisolone (30 mg/kg/day, 1 to 3 times). In the biopsy examination, diagnosis by hematoxylin and eosin staining and findings specific to rejection within 6 h were confirmed by immunostaining of frozen sections. For histological diagnosis, we stained the apoptosis-related proteins such as FasL and surface antigens of B cells, T cells, and NK cells in each case. Steroid pulse therapy was conducted following

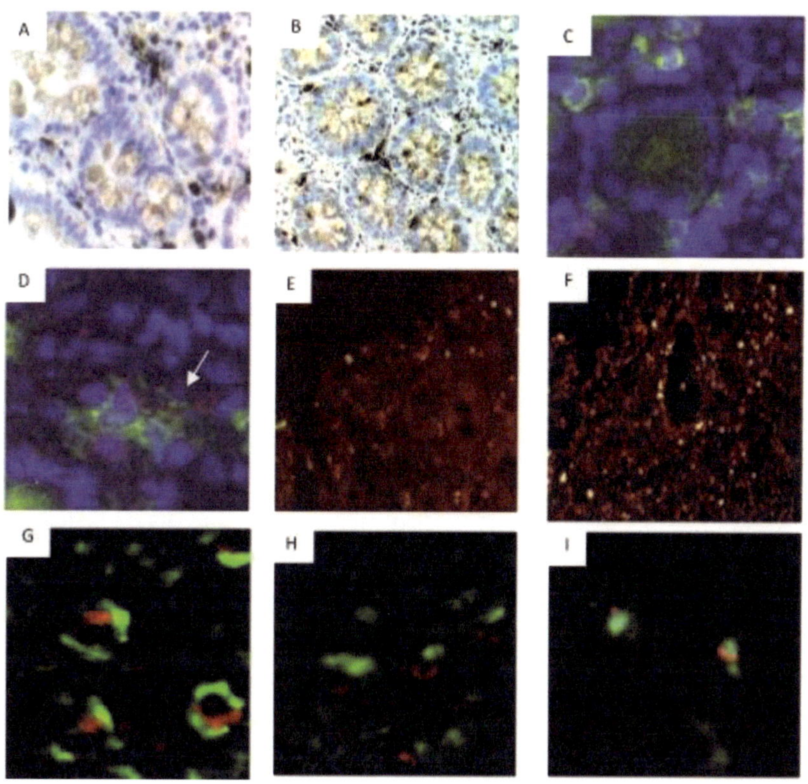

Figure 4.
Immunofluorescent staining of natural killer T cells in the intestinal allograft. Immunostaining of an intestinal allograft. Green signal, FITC and red signal, phycoerythrin [PE]. Nuclei are stained with DAPI (blue). Brown signal was visualized with DAB. (A) TCRVα24 (200×) and (B) TCRβ11 (200×). (C, D) TCRVα24 (green) and IL-4 (red) (IL-4 positive iNKT is indicated by an arrow). The observation magnification is 200× in both cases. (E, F) TCRVα24 (red) and TUNEL (green). (E) TUNEL+ (apoptotic) TCRVα24 + iNKT cells are observed at the onset of ACR (100×) and (F) 48 h after the onset of ACR (100×). Doubly stained cells were increased 48 h after the onset of ACR. (G) CD1d^{+} dendritic cells. CD1d and CD11c were stained green and red, respectively. (H) TCRVα24 stained iNKT cells (red) and CD1d stained dendritic cells (green). (I) FasL+ (green) TCRVα24+ (red) iNKT cells. The observation magnification is 400 x in (G)-(I).”

detecting the immunological activation with the appearance of FasL-positive T/NKT cells and apoptotic bodies in the lamina propria. The treatment substantially prevented the progression of the crypt apoptosis [17, 18, 21, 22].

5. Cytokine production in the intestinal allograft

5.1 NKT cells and cytokines

NKT cells are resident in the large bowel and increase in number in the colorectal cancer tissue [26]. The NKT cells have a limited T cell repertoire, and the restricted types are called invariant types of NKT (iNKT) cells. During the onset of intestinal rejection, the α chain 24 (TCRVα24) and β chain 11 (TCRVβ11) on iNKT cells are positively stained (**Figure 4A** and **B**) [17]. iNKT cells are mainly involved in innate immunity against glycolipids with the assistance of CD1d + dendritic cells [27]. Since iNKT cells are not identified in the small intestine of healthy donors before transplantation, this finding to be an indicator of ACR [17, 28].

Th1 cytokines, such as interferon-gamma (IFN-γ), generally act on the differentiation of CTLs, which promote rejection, while Th2 cytokines may suppress ACR of SBT. TCRVα24 (+) invariant NKT (iNKT) cells are positive for interleukin 4 (IL-4) in allografts of the intestine during rejection (**Figure 4C** and **D**) [8]. The apoptosis of iNKT cells are observed at the onset of rejection (**Figure 4E** and **F**), indicating that a part of apoptotic cells in the lamina propria are iNKT cells (**Figure 2**, lower right). CD1d+ dendritic cells are detected during the rejection process at the same time that the rejection progressed (**Figure 4G** and **H**). The involvement of iNKT cells in the rejection reaction has been discussed previously, and there is also an experimental report regarding their involvement in tolerance [29, 30]. However, the involvement of iNKT cells in rejection has not yet become apparent [31]. Furthermore, the mechanism by which the expression of IL-4 is directly involved in mucosal immune regulation remains unclear. However, IL-4 may suppress the action of CTLs that cause rejection. On the other hand, iNKT cells expressed FasL, indicating that they are activated in ACR (**Figure 4I**).

In addition, increased IL-5 production is also observed at the onset of rejection. IL-5 promotes eosinophil differentiation and chemotaxis [32]. This increase in production may explain the large number of eosinophils infiltrating the mucosa at the time of rejection [17]. Conventional T cells and iNKT cells may secrete IL-5 [17]. The role of eosinophils in rejection has often been debated [33] and there is a discussion on whether eosinophils may be the target of rejection therapy [34]. An increase in the rejection of eosinophils has also been reported in the transplanted liver [35]. In the small intestine, the presence of the mucosal immune system may further complicate the graft's immunological environment. Increased eosinophils, however, are histologically detectable and may provide useful information for the diagnosis of rejection, even in small bowel transplant grafts [5]. As a result of an imbalance in mucosal immunity, excess production of IL-4 and IL-5 may damage the mucosal epithelium. The administration of immunosuppressive drugs acts on iNKT cells in addition to cytotoxic T cells. Therefore, the distribution of immunocompetent lymphocytes in the mucosa is disturbed, and the treatment protocol should be developed further.

6. Histological tolerance of the intestinal allograft

Finally, we reviewed a case of histological tolerance reported [25]. This case involves a transplant in a 4-year-old male patient who had short bowel syndrome and previously underwent a living small bowel transplant from his mother who was in her twenties. The patient underwent a small intestinal biopsy 2–3 times per week for one month. Immunological analysis was performed using CD3, CD4, CD8, CD20, CD56, CD79a, perforin, granzyme B, FasL, Fas, and TUNEL staining. No severe rejection with an increase in FasL-positive T cells was detected. The maximum level of CRP, an inflammation marker, was 1.0 (mg/10^{-1} L) at POD67. In situ hybridization was performed using a Y-chromosome probe to evaluate rejection or tolerance for evaluation of the immunologic stability of the graft and chimerization [36], which comprises multiplex staining with a CD3 fluorescent substance, for monitoring allografts. **Figure 5** shows photographs of the graft 5 years after transplantation. A part of native T lymphocytes were replaced with Y-chromosome positive T lymphocytes from a male patient. This patient has been living for longer than ten years without any clinical symptoms, such as rejection, and is likely one of the first cases of operational tolerance.

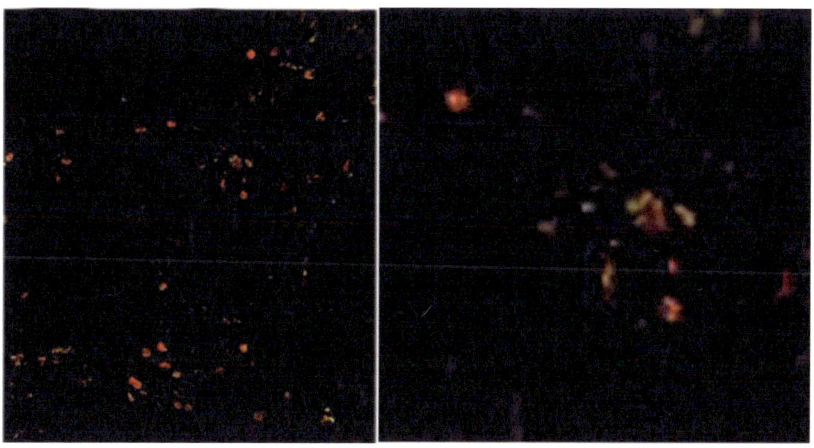

Figure 5.
Combined in situ hybridization of lymphocytes with the Y-chromosome probe (red: PE) and CD3-lymphocytic immunohistochemistry (green: FITC). The photos show the double-stained T cells carrying the Y-chromosomal investigation, indicating the male-donor derived lymphocytes in the female-derived intestinal allograft. Left (100×) and right (400×). The nuclei were stained red, indicating Y-chromosome positivity.

7. Conclusion

Early diagnosis of rejection of the transplanted small intestine is essential to facilitate the initiation of therapy that interferes with rejection progression. In addition to crypt apoptosis, apoptotic bodies in the lamina propria is considered useful for diagnosis. Furthermore, iNKT cell infiltration was another characteristic finding. Since histologic features of ACR have been studied extensively. Of note in future diagnoses are the issues of humoral and chronic rejection.

Appendices and nomenclature

ACR	acute cellular rejection
CMV	cytomegalovirus
CRP	C-reactive protein
CTL	cytotoxic T lymphocyte
EBV	Epstein–Barr virus

FasL	Fas ligand
FITC	fluorescein isothiocyanate
iNKT cells	invariant natural killer T cells
IL-4	interleukin 4
IL-5	interleukin 5
NKT cells	natural killer T cells
SBT	small bowel transplantation
TUNEL	terminal deoxynucleotidyl transferase dUTP nick end labeling

Author details

Tatsuaki Tsuruyama[1,2]

1 Department of Drug and Discovery Medicine, Pathology Division, Graduate School of Medicine, Kyoto University, Kyoto, Kyoto Prefecture, Japan

2 Tazuke-Kofukai Medical Institute, Kitano Hospital, Osaka, Osaka Prefecture, Japan

*Address all correspondence to: tatsuakitsuruyama@gmail.com

IntechOpen

© 2020 The Author(s). Licensee IntechOpen. This chapter is distributed under the terms of the Creative Commons Attribution License (http://creativecommons.org/licenses/by/3.0), which permits unrestricted use, distribution, and reproduction in any medium, provided the original work is properly cited.

References

[1] Pirenne J, Hoffman I, Miserez M, Coosemans W, Aerts R, Monbaliu D, et al. Selection criteria and outcome of patients referred to intestinal transplantation: an European center experience. Transplant Proc. 2006;**38**(6):1671-1672. Epub 2006/08/16. S0041-1345(06)00553-7 [pii]. doi: 10.1016/j.transproceed.2006.05.063. PubMed PMID: 16908242.

[2] Neuvonen MI, Kyrklund K, Lindahl HG, Koivusalo AI, Rintala RJ, Pakarinen MP. A population-based, complete follow-up of 146 consecutive patients after transanal mucosectomy for Hirschsprung disease. Journal of Pediatric Surgery. 2015;**50**(10):1653-1658. Epub 2015/03/19. PubMed PMID: 25783387. DOI: 10.1016/j.jpedsurg.2015.02.006

[3] Masetti M, Rodriguez MM, Thompson JF, Pinna AD, Kato T, Romaguera RL, et al. Multivisceral transplantation for megacystis microcolon intestinal hypoperistalsis syndrome. Transplantation. 1999;**68**(2):228-232 Epub 1999/08/10. PubMed PMID: 10440392

[4] Gerlach UA, Vrakas G, Reddy S, Baumgart DC, Neuhaus P, Friend PJ, et al. Chronic intestinal failure after Crohn disease: When to perform transplantation. JAMA Surgery. 2014;**149**(10):1060-1066. DOI: 10.1001/jamasurg.2014.1072 PubMed PMID: 25162284

[5] Pinna AD, Weppler D, Nery J, Ruiz P, Kato T, Khan F, et al. Intestinal transplantation at the University of Miami-five years of experience. Transplant Proc. 2000;**32**(6):1226-1227 Epub 2000/09/21. doi: S0041134500011994 [pii]. PubMed PMID: 10995922

[6] Tzakis AG, Kato T, Nishida S, Levi DM, Tryphonopoulos P, Madariaga JR, et al. Alemtuzumab (Campath-1H) combined with tacrolimus in intestinal and multivisceral transplantation. Transplantation. 2003;**75**(9):1512-1517 Epub 2003/06/07. doi: 10.1097/01.TP.0000060250.50591.39. PubMed PMID: 12792506

[7] Tzakis AG, Nery JR, Thompson J, Webb MG, Khan FA, Khan RT, et al. New immunosuppressive regimens in clinical intestinal transplantation. Transplant Proc. 1997;**29**(1-2):683-685 Epub 1997/02/01. PubMed PMID: 9123479

[8] Reyes J. Intestinal transplantation for children with short bowel syndrome. Seminars in Pediatric Surgery. 2001;**10**(2):99-104 Epub 2001/05/01. doi: S105585860100021X [pii]. PubMed PMID: 11329611

[9] Avitzur Y, Grant D. Intestine transplantation in children: update 2010. Pediatr Clin North Am. 2010;57(2):415-431, table of contents. Epub 2010/04/08. doi: S0031-3955(10)00020-9 [pii]. 10.1016/j.pcl.2010.01.019. PubMed PMID: 20371045

[10] Wu T, Abu-Elmagd K, Bond G, Nalesnik MA, Randhawa P, Demetris AJ. A schema for histologic grading of small intestine allograft acute rejection. Transplantation. 2003;**75**(8):1241-1248. Epub 2003/04/30. DOI: 10.1097/01.TP.0000062840.49159.2F PubMed PMID: 12717210

[11] Ruiz P, Takahashi H, Delacruz V, Island E, Selvaggi G, Nishida S, et al. International grading scheme for acute cellular rejection in small-bowel transplantation: single-center experience. Transplant Proc. 2010;**42**(1):47-53 Epub 2010/02/23. S0041-1345(09)01782-5 [pii] doi: 10.1016/j.transproceed.2009.12.026. PubMed PMID: 20172279.

[12] Ruiz P, Bagni A, Brown R, Cortina G, Harpaz N, Magid MS, et al. Histological criteria for the identification of acute cellular rejection in human small bowel allografts: results of the pathology workshop at the VIII International Small Bowel Transplant Symposium. Transplant Proc. 2004;**36**(2):335-337. Epub 2004/03/31. DOI: 10.1016/j.transproceed.2004.01.079 S0041134504000995 [pii]. PubMed PMID: 15050150

[13] Charles J, Di Domizio J, Salameire D, Bendriss-Vermare N, Aspord C, Muhammad R, et al. Characterization of circulating dendritic cells in melanoma: Role of CCR6 in plasmacytoid dendritic cell recruitment to the tumor. The Journal of Investigative Dermatology. 2010;**130**(6):1646-1656. DOI: 10.1038/jid.2010.24 PubMed PMID: 20220766

[14] Kubal CA, Pennington C, Fridell J, Ekser B, Muhaylov P, Mangus R. Challenges with Intestine and Multivisceral Re-Transplantation: Importance of Timing of Re-Transplantation and Optimal Immunosuppression. Ann Transplant. 2018;23:98-104. Epub 2018/02/07. doi: 10.12659/aot.908052. PubMed PMID: 29402878; PubMed Central PMCID: PMCPMC6248276.

[15] Koo J, Dawson DW, Dry S, French SW, Naini BV, Wang HL. Allograft biopsy findings in patients with small bowel transplantation. Clinical Transplantation. 2016;**30**(11):1433-1439. Epub 2016/11/03. PubMed PMID: 27582272. DOI: 10.1111/ctr.12836

[16] Jiang JW, Ren ZG, Lu HF, Zhang H, Li A, Cui GY, et al. Optimal immunosuppressor induces stable gut microbiota after liver transplantation. World J Gastroenterol. 2018;24(34):3871-3883. Epub 2018/09/20. doi: 10.3748/wjg.v24.i34.3871. PubMed PMID: 30228781; PubMed Central PMCID: PMCPMC6141331.

[17] Tsuruyama T, Fujimoto Y, Yonekawa Y, Miyao M, Onodera H, Uemoto S, et al. Invariant natural killer T cells infiltrate intestinal allografts undergoing acute cellular rejection. Transpl Int. 2012;25(5):537-544. Epub 2012/03/03. doi: 10.1111/j.1432-2277.2012.01450.x. PubMed PMID: 22380521.

[18] Tsuruyama T, Okamoto S, Fujimoto Y, Yoshizawa A, Yoshitoshi E, Egawa H, et al. Histology of intestinal allografts: Lymphocyte apoptosis and phagocytosis of lymphocytic apoptotic bodies are diagnostic findings of acute rejection in addition to crypt apoptosis. The American Journal of Surgical Pathology. 2013;**37**(2):178-184. DOI: 10.1097/PAS.0b013e31826393fe PubMed PMID: 23026933

[19] Tsuruyama T. Histopathology of intestinal transplant rejections. SOJ immunol. 2016;**4**(1):1-7

[20] Baulies A, Angelis N, Li VSW. Hallmarks of intestinal stem cells. Development. 2020;147(15). Epub 2020/08/05. doi: 10.1242/dev.182675. PubMed PMID: 32747330.

[21] Yoshitoshi EY, Yoshizawa A, Ogawa E, Kaneshiro M, Takada N, Okamoto S, et al. The challenge of acute rejection in intestinal transplantation. Pediatric Surgery International 2012;28(8):855-859. doi: 10.1007/s00383-012-3110-x. PubMed PMID: 22760434.

[22] Fujimoto Y, Uemoto S, Inomata Y, Egawa H, Fujita S, Kawanami T, et al. Small bowel transplantation using grafts from living-related donors. Two case reports. Transpl Int. 2000;13 Suppl 1:S179-S184. Epub 2000/12/09. PubMed PMID: 11111992.

[23] Krams SM, Hayashi M, Fox CK, Villanueva JC, Whitmer KJ, Burns W,

et al. CD8+ cells are not necessary for allograft rejection or the induction of apoptosis in an experimental model of small intestinal transplantation. J Immunol. 1998;160(8):3673-3680. Epub 1998/04/29. PubMed PMID: 9558067.

[24] McDiarmid SV, Farmer DG, Kuniyoshi JS, Robert M, Khadavi A, Shaked A, et al. Perforin and granzyme B. Cytolytic proteins up-regulated during rejection of rat small intestine allografts. Transplantation. 1995;59(5):762-766. Epub 1995/03/15. PubMed PMID: 7886805.

[25] Tsuruyama T. Histological image of transplanted small intestine. Japanese Journal of Pediatric Surgery. 2013;45(7):711-715. (In Japanese)

[26] Tachibana T, Onodera H, Tsuruyama T, Mori A, Nagayama S, Hiai H, et al. Increased intratumor Valpha24-positive natural killer T cells: a prognostic factor for primary colorectal carcinomas. Clin Cancer Res. 2005;11(20):7322-7327. Epub 2005/10/26. doi: 11/20/7322 [pii]. 10.1158/1078-0432.CCR-05-0877. PubMed PMID: 16243803.

[27] van Dieren JM, van der Woude CJ, Kuipers EJ, Escher JC, Samsom JN, Blumberg RS, et al. Roles of CD1d-restricted NKT cells in the intestine. Inflamm Bowel Dis. 2007;13(9):1146-1152. Epub 2007/05/04. doi: 10.1002/ibd.20164. PubMed PMID: 17476670.

[28] Tsuruyama T, Aini W. The Roles of Invariant NKT Cells in Bowel Immunity — Suppression of Tumor Progression and Rejection of Intestinal Transplants. 2014. doi: 10.5772/57588.

[29] Chu X, Kilpatrick E, Xiao X, Liu W, Demirci G, Exley M, et al. Islet allograft tolerance in the absence of invariant natural killer T cells. Clinical Immunology 2011;141(3):268-272. doi: 10.1016/j.clim.2011.09.003. PubMed PMID: 21996456; PubMed Central PMCID: PMC3221878.

[30] Brossay L, Chioda M, Burdin N, Koezuka Y, Casorati G, Dellabona P, et al. CD1d-mediated recognition of an alpha-galactosylceramide by natural killer T cells is highly conserved through mammalian evolution. Journal of Experimental Medicine. 1998;188(8):1521-1528. PubMed PMID: ISI:000076620100014.

[31] Vasan S, Tsuji M. A double-edged sword: The role of NKT cells in malaria and HIV infection and immunity. Seminars in Immunology 2010;22(2): 87-96. doi: 10.1016/j.smim.2009.11.001. PubMed PMID: 19962909; PubMed Central PMCID: PMC3603358.

[32] Rozenberg P, Reichman H, Zab-Bar I, Itan M, Pasmanik-Chor M, Bouffi C, et al. CD300f:IL-5 cross-talk inhibits adipose tissue eosinophil homing and subsequent IL-4 production. Sci Rep. 2017;7(1):5922. Epub 2017/07/21. doi: 10.1038/s41598-017-06397-4. PubMed PMID: 28725048; PubMed Central PMCID: PMCPMC5517555.

[33] Bush JW, Mohammad S, Melin-Aldana H, Kagalwalla AF, Arva NC. Eosinophilic density in graft biopsies positive for rejection and blood eosinophil count can predict development of post-transplant digestive tract eosinophilia. Pediatric Transplantation 2016;20(4):540-551. Epub 2016/02/27. doi: 10.1111/petr.12693. PubMed PMID: 26917244.

[34] Kers J, Florquin S. Eosinophil-targeted therapy: Not the panacea for antibody-mediated rejection? American Journal of Transplantation 2013;13(10):2522-2523. Epub 2013/08/08. doi: 10.1111/ajt.12402. PubMed PMID: 23919601.

[35] Krenzien F, Keshi E, Splith K, Griesel S, Kamali K, Sauer IM, et al.

Diagnostic Biomarkers to Diagnose Acute Allograft Rejection After Liver Transplantation: Systematic Review and Meta-Analysis of Diagnostic Accuracy Studies. Front Immunol. 2019;10:758. Epub 2019/04/30. doi: 10.3389/fimmu.2019.00758. PubMed PMID: 31031758; PubMed Central PMCID: PMCPMC6470197.

[36] Aini W, Miyagawa-Hayashino A, Tsuruyama T, Hashimoto S, Sumiyoshi S, Ozeki M, et al. Telomere shortening and karyotypic alterations in hepatocytes in long-term transplanted human liver allografts. Transpl Int. 2012;25(9):956-966. doi: 10.1111/j.1432-2277.2012.01523.x. PubMed PMID: 22775391.

Chapter 6

Regulatory T Cells in the Mosaic of Liver Transplantation Tolerance

Velislava Terzieva, Yordanka Uzunova, Radosvet Gornev and Lubomir Spassov

Abstract

The success of transplantation depends on multiple factors, but the establishment of immune tolerant milieu is of critical importance. Hepatic environment consists of different cellular populations with prominent capacity to tolerate a huge range of antigens. Among them, regulatory T cells (Tregs) play an important role. They control the strength of immune reactions against non-self antigens and were shown to have an impact on the establishment of immune tolerance in the post-transplantation period. Furthermore, they impact a particular state after transplantation – operational tolerance. The abundant data show that Tregs might be manipulated, which suggests their further implementation as a treatment strategy. Tregs are also a very attractive target as a biomarker in the monitoring of post-transplantation period. Here, we review the particular role of Tregs among the broad spectrum of immune tolerance mechanisms of the liver in the light of the current directions of medical research.

Keywords: liver transplantation, regulatory T cells, immune tolerance, biomarker, operational tolerance

1. Introduction

Transplantation is the most beneficial approach to treat diseases, manifested by irreversible changes of the liver parenchyma. The success of transplantation depends on both the surgical operation and the development of an immune tolerant milieu in the post-transplantation period. In solid organ transplantation, the immunological mechanisms that are naturally dedicated to the defense from foreign antigens (microbial, viral etc.), are directed towards HLA (MHC) molecules and allo-antigens of the graft. This powerful immune reaction may destroy the graft and compromise the beneficial effect of the transplant. In the routine clinical practice, the control of effector immune function is achieved through immune suppressive therapy. However, in kidney and liver transplantation a spontaneous development of immune tolerance where a particular T cells subset – regulatory T cells (Tregs) is supposed to play important role [1].

Thus, recent achievements in transplantation research motivate the focus on the immunological mechanisms in two directions. From one side, this is the continuous investigation on new and more relevant biomarkers for the monitoring of the post-transplantation period and prediction of graft rejection. From the other side, is the need of new therapeutic opportunities that might be influenced by the scientific research on the fine immune mechanisms [2].

IntechOpen

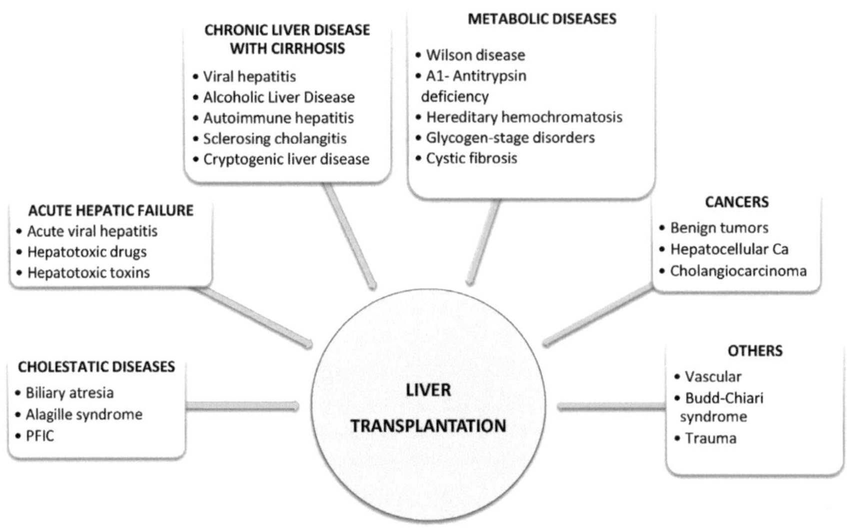

Figure 1.
Principal medical conditions that require liver transplantation.

Studies on Tregs are particularly intense in the field of transplantology precisely in connection with their suppressive function. Lots of data in the literature on their behavior in transplantation of solid organs as well as stem cells is present. While in kidney, heart and other transplants already have outlined trends in the dynamics and even the therapeutic application of Tregs [3], the situation with liver transplantation (LT) is more special.

Patients with life-limiting liver disease, which may present in the form of acute liver failure, end-stage chronic liver disease, hepatic malignancy, or inborn metabolic disorders need LT - liver function is heavily impaired as a result of irreversible morphological changes (**Figure 1**).

Whatever the cause, the outcome of liver transplantation depends on three main factors: the clinical approach, the immune characteristics of the liver, and the therapeutic provision of immunological tolerance.

2. Clinical aspects of liver transplantation

From a clinical point of view, the outcome of transplantation depends on the general condition of the recipient (MELD score in adults and PELD score in children) before surgery and the quality of the graft, surgical technique, postoperative care, immunosuppressive therapy. The operation is one of the largest in volume and complexity in surgery in general. Most often in Europe and the United States the so-called "standard" LT is performed, in which an entire organ is transplanted - whole liver graft. Deceased liver transplantation (DLT) is not common in Asia and part of a living donor organ is used [4, 5].

In deceased, an organ donation is possible when the graft is from a donor who has been registered as brain dead (brain dead donor) and donation after cardiac death.

Liver transplantation from a living donor (LDLT) offers some advantages over cadaveric donation: determining the time of the operation, the graft is from a healthy person and is in optimal condition, the cold ischemia time is shortened. It is suitable for children due to the possibility of precise selection of the graft in accordance with the patient's weight. Choosing a donor candidate is sometimes difficult due to the presence of arterial variations combined with additional abnormalities in other vessels and the biliary tract [6]. LDLT is suitable in cases of rare diseases in patients under 1 year of age. Of the pediatric liver transplantations performed at Lozenets University Hospital, about 65.5% of the patients are in this age group, and between 10 and 18 years of age they are significantly fewer [7].

Another type is domino transplantation, but it is rarely performed. Indication for it is Familial amyloid polyneuropathy (FAP). The disease affects extrahepatic organs and liver function is preserved. This allows the liver of the FAP patient to be given to another patient, from whom (in turn) receives the damaged organ (domino effect) [8]. The main requirement for the FAP recipient is to be over 55–60 years old, in order to minimize the risk of developing the disease.

Partial transplantation is performed as a matter of urgency in two specific situations. The first is in acute liver failure, in order to support the damaged organ until its recovery. The graft is then removed and the immunosuppressive therapy is stopped. The second case is in patients with congenital functional or metabolic disorders that affect the liver. Implantation of the partial graft preserves its own organ, corrects metabolic abnormalities and does not require whole liver transplantation [9]. In both situations, the transplant can be orthotropic or heterotropic.

A variant of the partial transplantation is the split-transplant, in which the two lobes are distributed between two recipients. In recent years, due to the increased number of patients on the waiting list and the small number of potential donors, the technique of split-liver transplantation has been applied in which in vivo /in situ or ex-vivo/ex-situ the liver is divided into two parts - right for adult transplantation and left for pediatric transplantation. In some cases, it is possible to use the split-technique for transplantation of two adults. It is preferable to perform split-LT in-vivo, which reduces the risk of biliary complications, hemorrhage and significantly reduces the cold ischemia time of the graft [4, 5]. The main condition is the ratio between the weight of the graft and the patient, which must be at least 0.8% [4, 10]. The aim is to ensure the long-term vital functions of the recipient.

The complexity of the operation creates preconditions for the occurrence of complications during and after the operation. In the postoperative period, the leading are vascular and biliary complications, stenosis of the anastomosis, risk of infection and others.

In the long term, the outcome of transplantation depends largely on the establishment of optimal post-transplant immune tolerance. Here the immunological features of the liver, which distinguish it from other organs, play a significant role.

3. Tolerogenic milieu of the liver

The liver is a metabolic organ with a principal role of the detoxification and nutrient storage, but also protein synthesis and production of biochemicals required for the digestion and growth.

Without a doubt, the liver is also an important element of the immune system. A broad range of parts of innate and adaptive immunity is synthesized inside like acute-phase proteins, cytokines, complement components etc. Indeed, the cells that populate the liver encompass not only those with metabolic function. A great variety of immune cells are found in the parenchyma. Liver sinusoidal endothelial cells (LSECs), Kupffer cells, dendritic cells, hepatic stellate cells (HSCs), natural killer (NK) cells, NKT cells and T cells are present in the liver interstitium. In addition, hepatic cells express surface receptors immanent for the innate immunity [11]. Altogether, they participate in the establishment of a particular milieu that from one hand tolerates a broad range of gut-derived antigens continuously passing across and on the other hand, retain the capacity to set up an immune response against pathogens like bacteria and viruses.

The questions of how this community maintains an immunotolerant environment to nutritional antigens, provide effector response to pathogens and guarantee liver transplantation are of particular interest. Moreover, the graft rejection is relatively rare in LT as compared to other SOT.

The combination of particular anatomy, variety of cells, specific expression of HLA molecules [12] and sustained antigenic stimulation makes the liver a unique immunologic structure. The blood delivered by vena portae is rich in alimentary and other antigens, which in fact are tolerated by the healthy liver. Indeed, the basal levels of pro- and anti-inflammatory cytokines are constant, but change under pathologic conditions in etiology-dependent manner [13–15].

The liver primarily is a metabolic organ and this function significantly impacts its immunologic reactivity. The metabolism of carbohydrates and lipids has a particular impact. Absorbed by hepatocytes, they are collected as glycogen and lipoproteins. Further on, cholesterol, triglycerides and other intermediate metabolites can trigger TLR signalization and inflammasome activation. The final result is the increased pro-inflammatory cytokines secretion followed by the initiation of different pathologic phenomena, liver fibrosis for example [16]. Another example demonstrates that metabolic variations in hepatocytes during hepatitis B and C infection can raise viral replication [17, 18].

Together with hepatocytes, dendritic cells and macrophages also participate in the hepatic cytokine regulation. The oxidative phosphorylation may switch to anaerobic glycolysis (effect Warburg) leading to stimulation of pro-inflammatory mediators synthesis [19, 20]. Succinate dehydrogenase can additionally influence the cytokine balance. Its high levels may activate Hypoxia induced factor-1 (HIF-1) and production of IL-1β, thus providing evidence for the direct communication between the cellular metabolism and inflammatory response [21]. IL-1β per se is an important player in the control of homeostasis by regulating sleep, feeding, temperature in healthy conditions [22]. In pathologic situations, IL-1β is a critical mediator of the inflammatory response through processing of pro-IL-1β by Caspase-1 via inflammasome [23, 24]. Other mechanisms can be also involved in the cleavage of pro-IL-1β into biologically active IL-1b. Among them are serine proteases-neutrophil elastase, proteinase 3, cathepsin G in neutrophils [25–27] and the spontaneous release of IL-1β following pyroptosis and necroptosis [28]. Not surprisingly, IL-1β levels were found increased in other, relatively frequent medical conditions like NAFLD [29].

4. Tolerogenic properties of liver cells

Hepatic cells represent a heterogeneous population where different liver residents have their own tolerogenic approach (**Figure 2**).

4.1 Hepatocytes

Parenchymal hepatocytes are the major population in the liver. Although being involved in metabolism, toxin neutralization and glycogen synthesis, they function also as immune cells by expressing immune-associated molecules like pattern recognition receptors (PRRs), adhesion and major histocompatibility complex (MHC) molecules [30, 31]. The latter permit hepatocytes to act as antigen-presenting cells for CD8+ T cells and to trigger their activation and proliferation [32]. However, the particular hepatic environment does not ensure the required survival factors

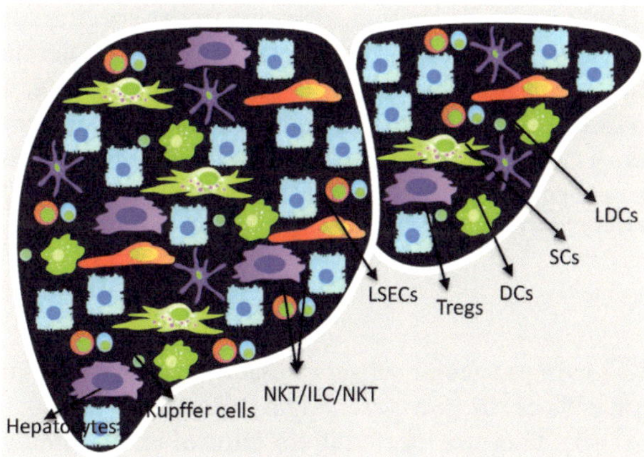

Cell type	Tolerogenic capacity
Hepatocytes	Expression of PRRs, MHC molecules, antigen presentation, , induction of Tregs
Kupffer cells	Receptors for complement and antibodies, TLRs, cytokines
Liver Sinusoidal Endothelial Cells	Expression of TLRs, RIGs and B7-H1, antigen presentation,
Stellate Cells (SCs)	Antigen presentation, PD-L1, B7-H7, Fas/Fas-L expression, induction of Tregs
Liver Dendritic Cells (LDCs)	Generation of Tregs, immunosuppressive cytokines
NKT/ILC/NKT	Limited response to stimulation vie TCR, weak suppressive potential
Regulatory T cells (Tregs)	Production of suppressive cytokines, expression of inhibitory molecules, Potential to be introduced as immune therapy after transplantation

Figure 2.
The mosaic of tolerogenic cells in the liver. On the table below are shown main tolerogenic mechanisms, employed by every population.

for CD8+ cells and they rapidly undergo activation-induced apoptosis [33]. Interestingly, the inflammatory response can be accompanied by the expression of MHC class II molecules followed by antigen presentation to CD4+ T cells [34, 35]. Depending on the differentiation status of helper cells, they may undergo Th2 differentiation of uncommitted CD4 T cells, or abrogated ability of previously differentiated Th1 to secrete interferon-γ, and finally - switch of CD4 + T effector cells towards induced regulatory T cells (FoxP3 + CD25+) [33, 36] . Ergo, liver parenchymal cells have substantial tolerogenic potential directed to both CD4+ and CD8+ T cells. Whether all would be launch together or not need to be elucidated.

4.2 Liver sinusoidal endothelial cells

Liver sinusoidal endothelial cells (LSECs) are an important part of the reticuloendothelial system. They are highly specialized and form the lining of the hepatic sinusoids. Their characteristic morphology (abundant fenestrae) and the permanent exposition to the blood flow permit them to filter out blood antigens. From an immunological viewpoint LSECs are liver-resident antigen-presenting cells that might be considered as bridge between the innate and adaptive immunity. It is evidenced by the expression of TLRs and RIGs, which under stimulation, turn on the production of proinflammatory cytokines, upregulation of costimulatory molecules and release of cytokines, that affect T cells [13, 37]. In parallel, LSECs may present antigens to T cells although not being professional APCs as shown by the expression of MHC class I on the LSECs surface [15]. The question about MHC class II expression is still not well clarified, although under specific conditions, LSECs may present antigens to CD4+ T cells inducing immune tolerance [38] . LSEC actively participate in the induction of tolerance. For example, in naïve CD8+ T cells, the cognate interaction triggers the expression of co-inhibitory B7-H1 but not the co-stimulatory CD80/86 molecules exclusively on LSEC but not DC, which together with increased costimulation via CD28 is critical for the induction of CD8+ T cell tolerance by LSEC [39].

4.3 Kupffer cells

Kupffer cells (KCs) are particular subset of macrophages, settled in the liver. They represent appr. 35% of the non-parenchymal liver cells and 90% of all tissue macrophages [40]. They are located in the sinusoids, thus being systematically exposed to gut-derived antigens, circulating immune cells and pathogens. The principle function of KCs is pathogen killing. However, KCs are armed with scavenger receptors, TLRs, complement receptors and antibody receptors, secrete cytokines and chemokines and express broad range of receptor molecules [41]. Thus, KCs not only participate in antimicrobial killing, but also are an active player in the immune network. Their primary function is the antigen presentation. They express MHC class I and class II molecules which together with other costimulatory molecules activate T cells. In healthy conditions, KCs promote immune tolerance in several ways – lower expression of MHC class II, B7–1, B7–2, CD40, PD-1/PD-1 L and possible involvement of IL-10, nitric oxide, TGF-b [38, 42]. Other mechanisms include the ability of KCs to absorb and clear alloreactive antibodies in liver transplantation [43]. Conversely, when stimulated (through TLRs for ex.), KCs become potent activators of T cells and NK cells [44]. In animal models, depletion of graft Kupffer cells was beneficial for the graft acceptance [45]. The double sword performance of KCs needs to be investigated in details, especially in humans. In any case, the current knowledge clearly indicates the KCs impact heavily on the reactivity of the liver immune system.

4.4 Stellate cells

Hepatic Stellate cells (HSCs) are another subset with immune function. This relatively small population (5–10% of liver parenchymal cells) resides in the space of Disse and is primarily involved in the storage of retinoid droplets and vitamin A and regulation of blood flow in the sinusoids [32, 46, 47]. In the intact liver, they are quiescent cells. Once activated, they differentiate to myofibroblast and participate in hepatic fibrosis pathogenesis [48]. The second direction of their function is the immunosuppression. Study in animals and humans show that they are effective antigen presenting cells with tolerogenic capacity because of the expression of PD-L1, B7-H7 and Fas/Fas-L pathways [49–51]. When activated, HSCs induce myeloid derived suppressor cells and Foxp3+ regulatory T cells by production of retinoic acid [52] In addition, they produce a broad range of cytokines, like TGF-b, IL-6 etc., and are able to respond to them, thus actively participate in the immune-mediated network in the liver [48].

4.5 Liver dendritic cells

Dendritic cells (DCs) are professional antigen-presenting cells. Following the antigen processing, they activate T cells and unlock the adaptive immune reaction. The liver-resident DCs are distinct population as compared to blood DCs. While DCs expressing CD1c and CD14 represent 95% of blood DCs, in liver they are 70%

and those expressing CD141 increase up to 30% [53]. It is still unclear in details how these cells contribute to the development of immune tolerance. Although some evidences that DCs may enhance graft rejection by increase of CD80 and CD86 expression [54, 55], the depletion of donor DCs is followed by graft rejection [56]. The investigations of Bamboat et al. demonstrate that liver DCs generate more suppressive $CD4^{+}CD25^{+}FoxP3+$ T regulatory cells and IL-4-producing Th2 cells via an IL-10-dependent mechanism [57]. Another particular feature of LDCs is their low endocytosis capacity and weak capacity to stimulate T cells. Conversely, they produce high levels of the immunosuppressive IL-10 [58, 59]. The comparison with their splenic match reveal important differences: lower secretion of type I interferons, "lipid-based dichotomy" – lipid contents dependent antigen presentation, plasmacytoid DC ($B220^{+}$) account for 19% of liver DC, but only 5% of spleen DC [60–62].

4.6 NK, ILC cells and NKT cells

Natural killer cells represent 30–50% of hepatic lymphocytes [63]. They differ from conventional NK cells and are closer to innate lymphoid cells (ILCs). In mouse they are closer to ILCs1, because of the expression of NK1.1 (CD161), CD69, CD49a NKp46, TRAIL. Both in mouse and human, these cells express CD49a and CD69 and secrete IFN-g and TNFa, but have weak suppressive capacity [64]. The third subset NKT cells are well presented in the liver. Different subsets are differentially presented in mice and humans, but have similar function – support immune homeostasis, control autoimmune reactions and immune responses to microbial and viral infections and cancer [65]. Of particular interest are invariant NKT and mucosal-associated invariant T cells (MAIT). They are $CD3^{+}CD4^{-}CD161^{+}V\alpha7.2^{+}$ cells and have robust IFN-g and granzymes B response to inflammatory signal, but limited responsiveness when stimulated directly via TCR [66, 67].

Therefore, the proper hepatic cells have dual function. On one hand they are involved in metabolic processes in the liver and on the other – they participate in immune-mediated reactions per se and by carrying out the function of a bridge between biochemical reactions and immune pathways.

Hepatic cells interact with local immune cells and thus actively participate in the establishment of a sustained immune tolerant milieu. Zheng and Tian (2019) analyzing current data, highlight the death of effector cells and the "education" of regulatory cells as key processes leading to the development of liver tolerance. Additionally, they describe a broad spectrum of baseline immune mechanisms responsible for the state of hyporesponsiveness – clonal deletion, clonal anergy, clonal deviation, T cell dysfunction/exhaustion, education etc. [68].

5. Regulatory T cells – conditio sine qua non for liver transplantation tolerance

5.1 General characteristics of regulatory T cells

Regulatory T cells are considered as the effector cellular arm of immune tolerance. Since the first publication of Kojima (1976), there is a constantly growing interest towards Tregs – cellular properties and medical applications [69]. Along with their unique suppressive phenotype (CD25 + FoxP3 + CD4+ T cells) [68, 69], Tregs express broad range of molecules that mirror their affiliation to the population of T cells and are widely applied in research and medical practice. Similarly to conventional T cells, they may be differentiated as naïve and memory, based on the expression of CD45RA, recent thymic emigrants (CD31), activated (HLA-DR) etc. [70, 71]. Their trafficking is ensured by the expression of chemokine receptors [72, 73].

The hallmark of Tregs is the expression of the transcription factor FoxP3 [68]. It controls the transcription program of Tregs by regulating several genes – increases expression of *Il2ra* (CD25), *Ctla4* (CTLA-4), *Tnfrsf18* (GITR), but inhibits those of *Il2.* At the same time *Foxp3* is subject of a tight regulation, where STAT5 signaling pathway is probably of key importance [74–77]. One may say that this is as two step process, starting with the generation of $CD25^{hi,}$ but $FoxP3^{-}$ Tregs-precursors, followed by the induction of FoxP3 through cytokine/STAT5-dependant signals involving HDAC [74, 78, 79]. Blocking of JAK/STAT pathway downmodulates Foxp3 expression [80]. In addition, a group of studies indicate that the maintenance of Tregs suppressive function is dependent on the epigenetic regulation of foxp3 locus by the Polycomb repressive complex 2 (PRC2). PRC2 consists of four subunits, primarily of enhancer of zeste homolog 2 (EZH2), EED, SUZ12, and RbAp48, where EZH2 is of particular interest [81]. The function of EHZ2 differs among different T-cell populations, leading to variations in H3K27me3 levels and silenced genes. In FoxP3 negative cells, EZH2 deficiency is associated with autoimmune diseases, reduced number of Tregs and expansion of memory T cells [82, 83].

The origin of Tregs in periphery is still a hot topic. Clear evidences show that a subset of Tregs - thymic Tregs (tTregs), come directly from the thymus during the process of intrathymic maturation of T cells [84–86]. Their selection occurs predominantly in the medulla during the negative selection by the high-avidity interactions between mTECs and thymocytes [87, 88], although some studies indicate that the process starts earlier, in the cortex [89]. Under specific conditions, like increased concentration of TGF-β, hormonal changes or continuous antigenic stimulation, Tregs can arise from naïve CD4+ T cells in periphery – inducible Tregs (iTregs) [90–92].

5.2 Tregs are armed by different suppressive mechanisms

Independently of the origin, Tregs are powerful immune suppressors. Both subsets use several approaches to regulate the strength of the immune response. Roughly, they are based on the expression of particular molecules, secretion of cytokines and consumption of IL-2 and might be categorized as contact-dependent and contact-independent.

Early studies demonstrated that the contact-dependent way is effectuate by the constitutive expression of CD152 (CTLA-4) by Tregs [93, 94]. The engagement of CD80/CD86 pathway activates tryptophan catabolism and expression of indoleamin 2,3 dioxygenase (IDO) [95]. Another mechanism involves PD-1/PD-L1 [95]. It is effective both against autoreactive B cells [96] and T lymphocytes [97]. Dilek et al. using alloreactive human T cells and blocking antibodies, evidenced by live cell dynamic microscopy that CD28, CTLA-4, and PD-L1 differentially control velocity, motility and immune synapse formation in activated Teff versus Tregs [94]. Although natural, their expression on the Tregs surface is inducibly increased and ensures the negative regulation of different receptors mediated signaling cascades in the target cells [98, 99]. Thus, Tregs directly attenuate cellular proliferation and activation.

The second line is facilitated by the production of different soluble factors upon activation. Among them are the immunosuppressive cytokines IL-10, TGF-b [100, 101], IL-34 [102] and IL-35 [103, 104]; perforins and granzymes [105]. It should be also considered that Tregs are target of cytokines like the proinflammatory TNF-α. The exact effect needs to be precised because current data are controversial. The study of Valencia et al. evidenced that treatment with anti-TNF antibody (infliximab) increases FOXP3 mRNA and protein expression by $CD4^{+}CD25^{hi}$ Tregs and restored their suppressive function [106]. Later on, Chen et al. shows that upon in vitro activation with plate-bound anti-CD3 Ab and soluble anti-CD28 Ab, Foxp3 expression by highly purified mouse Tregs is markedly downregulated. TNF partially abrogates this effect and stabilizes Foxp3 expression as this effect of TNF can be blocked by anti-TNFR2 Ab, but not by anti-TNFR1 Ab [107, 108]. In any case, the role of TNF-a needs to be further investigated because TNF-a plays important role in the inflammatory reactions, where Tregs are expected to be also involved.

Upon activation, effector T cells produce IL-2, which stimulates T cells proliferation and the expansion of the immune response. At the same time, Tregs are distinguished by the their high expression of CD25 [109]. These facts suggest that Tregs need IL-2 to survive [110, 111]. Placed in an activated milieu, Tregs may compete with effector cells and as a result, decrease the levels of IL-2 in the environment. In fact, this is the third approach that Tregs apply to achieve a state of suppression [112, 113].

Regulatory T cells apply all of the above-mentioned approaches for the establishment of immune-tolerant milieu. Still, there are no evidences about the mechanism preferred by nTregs or iTregs. Similarly, despite the abundance of data, no specific mechanisms can be attributed to a particular pathologic condition. Probably, the modus operandi of Tregs depends on the finetuning of T-cell receptor-antigen recognition and interaction, the target cell characteristics and the cytokine spectrum in the surrounding milieu.

5.3 The impact of regulatory T cells on the operational tolerance

The establishment of immune tolerance after solid organ transplantation (SOT) is the key therapeutic challenge in the post-operative period. In most cases, it is induced by the continuous application of immunosuppressive therapy. However, in some patients, a discontinuation of the regimen arrives, due to infections, cancer etc. Surprisingly, in some cases changes in immunological parameters, indicating the development of a state of immune tolerance were found despite the lack of immune suppression. This particular situation is defined as operational tolerance and is characterized by the absence of any clinical and histological signs of rejection in therapy free patients [114]. The operational tolerance (OT) is reported after transplantation of different solid organs, but is frequent in LT [115, 116]. It is supposed that tolerogenic properties of the liver and residential lymphocytes play a key role in this process [117]. The exact mechanisms are not fully clarified, but the intensive research highlights that it depends on multiple factors. Among them are regulatory T cells, particular gene expression profile and serum levels of HLA-G.

Regulatory T cells are the first parameter associated with OT. In patients with spontaneous tolerance they are increased independently of the age of recipient [118]. According to the study of Koshiba et al., not only the proportion CD4 + CD25high + T cells was increased in the tolerant patients' peripheral lymphocytes and suppressed MLR specifically to the donor antigen, but also FOXP3 expressing cells were present within the tolerant liver [119]. Pons and colleagues describe sustained increase in CD4 + CD25+ and CD4 + $CD25^{hi}$ cells in patients with operational tolerance in comparison with non-OT patients in a bimonthly evaluation intervals until M16 [1].

Interestingly, in LT Tregs show a particular dynamic. In one of the earliest studies, pre-transplantation levels of Tregs were higher in patients than in controls. Lowest levels were observed at month 3 after Tx, followed by a relative increase at 12 months and at later time points [120].

The main question is why these cells are elevated in recipients? In fact, up to now reports discussing this topic in the literature are insufficient. The detailed study of Demirkiran and colleagues examined the presence and allosuppressive activity of CD4 + CD25 + Foxp3+ Tregs in perfusates of human liver grafts and monitored the cells presence in the circulation of recipients after liver Tx. The authors show an increased proportion of CD4 + CD25 + CTLA4+ T cells compared with healthy control blood. The increased percentages of Foxp3+ cells, which were negative for CD127, confirmed the enrichment of Tregs in perfusates. They suppressed proliferation and IFN-γ production of donor and recipient T cells. In vivo within the first weeks after Tx, up to 5% of CD4 + CD25 + CTLA4+ T cells in recipient blood were derived from the donor liver, indicating that a substantial number of donor Tregs detach from the liver graft during perfusion and continue to migrate into the recipient after Tx. These donor Tregs suppress the direct pathway alloresponses and may in vivo contribute to chimerism-associated tolerance early after liver Tx [121]. In a small number of patients, we found a pick in the percentage of Tregs at day 7 (D7) followed by a decrease until D30 being always around and above healthy controls values independently of the diagnosis or age. The simultaneous routine measurement of liver function laboratory parameters revealed that the increase in Tregs precedes albumin synthesis restoration [122]. In another study Baumann et al. evidence that the benign clinical course of subclinical rejection (SCR) compared to acute clinical rejection (ACR) is associated with intrahepatic T cell infiltration patterns showing less cytotoxic T cells and more CD4 + FOXP3+ Tregs. They demonstrate that in patients with SCR the pattern of infiltrating T cells is characterized by a stronger accumulation of CD4+ cells, an increasing CD4+/CD8+ ratio, and an increasing CD4+ forkhead box P3 (FOXP3) + regulatory T cell (Treg)/CD8+ ratio, which was not seen in acute clinical rejection. These intrahepatic T cell patterns were not reflected in the peripheral blood [123]. Cumulatively, these data suggest the presence of particular sort of cellular chimerism, associated with liver transplantation.

The chimerism is a specific phenomenon characterized by the presence of cells from one individual in another. Microchimerism is reported in hematopoietic stem cells transplantation as a result of migration of passenger lymphocytes from the graft into recipient and in pregnancy (foetus). In SOT, microchimerism is described in mice first [124]. Among multiple reports showing than donor mononuclear cells migrate from the graft in the recipient, Jonsson et al. find that the peak levels of chimerism are within the first 48 hours after transplantation and the range reaches 20% of total peripheral blood mononuclear cells [125, 126]. In a concise and very interesting review, Abrol and colleagues assume that increased expression of chemokines in the liver attracts alloreactive T cells that are subsequently destroyed by coming in contact with various liver cells inherently programmed towards tolerance induction [127]. Donor specific hypo-responsiveness, down regulation of T helper type I cytokine (IFN-γ) and no change in T helper type 2 cytokine (IL10) in the *in vitro* mixed lymphocyte reaction in recipients who achieved operational tolerance were also reported [128]. Indeed, this topic needs more studies directed to the detailed evaluation of different cellular subsets. Probably, Tregs might be part of passenger leucocytes or they might be secondary induced by the modified hepatic environment.

6. Other tolerogenic strategies

Tregs are not the only approach, involved in tolerance establishment in liver transplantation. Other cells also participate in by expressing particular molecules or changing their genetic pattern.

In 16 operationally tolerant liver recipients, 16 recipients requiring on-going immunosuppressive therapy, and 10 healthy individuals by microarray profiling Martinez-Llordella et al. identified a gene expression signature that could discriminate tolerant recipients from immunosuppression-dependent patients with high accuracy. This signature included genes encoding for γδ T-cell and NK receptors, and for proteins involved in cell proliferation arrest. In addition, tolerant recipients exhibited significantly greater numbers of circulating potentially regulatory T-cell subsets (CD4 + CD25+ T-cells and Vδ1+ T cells) than either non-tolerant patients or healthy individuals [129].

The human leucocyte antigen-G (HLA-G) is a non-classical HLA class I molecule with prominent tolerogenic properties. It inhibits cytotoxicity and proliferation, but stimulates the development of regulatory T cells. HLA-G is present as a membrane-associated form and a soluble one. Interestingly, the uptake of HLA-G by some resting but mostly in activated CD4 and CD8 T cells leads to the instant generation of a new type of regulatory cells that initially act through cell-surface molecules that they temporarily display but do not express themselves [130–132]. This mechanisms is defined as trogocytosis and seems to play important role for the establishment of immune tolerance [133]. Several groups provides evidences about the role of HLA-G in kidney and heart transplantation [134–136]. In healthy conditions in adults, HLA-G is weakly expressed in liver, but it might be transmitted through transendothelial migration and/or trogocytosis from circulating cells under particular circumstances like cytokines, hypoxia etc. [137–139]. In all cases, elevated levels of sHLA-G is associated with reduced risk of rejection and better survival [140, 141].

7. Clinical relevance of regulatory T cells for liver transplantation

Slowly, but without doubt, regulatory T cells are getting involved in the diagnostic process of many pathological conditions, expressed by deviations in immune tolerance – autoimmune [142, 143], tumors [144, 145], recurrent pregnancy loss [146, 147], primary immune deficiencies [110, 148] etc.

Current data indicate that Tregs have the potential to be a potential biomarker for the monitoring of the posttransplantation period [2]. Specifically, in liver transplanted patients Tregs are object of intensive research mostly because they are inherently involved in the operational tolerance and are part of natural liver toleragenic mechanisms. Despite the abundant data showing the benefit of Tregs determination during posttransplantation period, there are still many unresolved questions. Some of them are related to the definition of Tregs phenotype that should be used. Although identified as FoxP3 + CD4+ T cells, the expression of FoxP3 was demonstrated less informative than the promotore demethylation because it distinguishes true Tregs from transiently FOXP3+ activated T cells [149]. For diagnostic purposes, Tregs are often defined as CD127-CD25 + CD4+, but recent advances in the field showed a population CD25- [150], which is not fully characterized regarding CD127. Another direction that needs to be elucidated are Tregs in biopsies and peripheral blood. In Barcelona consensus (2016) several studies are shown with ambiguous results [151], that does not provide clear evidences for the relevance of Tregs measurement in posttransplantation period. The third direction is the significantly decreased expression of CD25 in relation to the immunosuppressive therapy and the consecutive inability to find out CD25^{hi}Treg cells in the periphery. Although Tregs are highly informative regarding the operational tolerance [152], the question is still unresolved and more studies are required to determine the value of Tregs in the monitoring of post-transplantation period.

It seems, that Tregs are more promising as a therapeutic approach for the control of immune activation and development of a state of immune tolerance. Early experimental studies demonstrated association between them and the delay in islet allograft rejection and long term survival [153, 154]. During last five years, together with other approaches [155], Tregs attract the medical interest in the field of GVHD and solid organ transplantation [156, 157]. Todo et al. in 2016 report phase I results clinical trial with ex vivo expanded recipient polyclonal Tregs in living kidney transplants. Despite variability in recipient's renal disease, the expansion protocol produced Tregs which met all release criteria, expressing >98% CD4 + CD25+ with <1% CD8+ and CD19+ contamination and > 80% FOXP3 expression with stable demethylation in the FOXP3 promoter. Within recipients, expanded Tregs amplified circulating Treg levels in a sustained manner. Clinically, all doses of Treg therapy tested were safe with no adverse infusion related side effects, infections or rejection events up to two years post-transplant [158]. Another study undertook a direct comparison of the *in vitro* and *in vivo* functional activities of the different memory and naïve Treg subpopulations showing that the naive Treg is the Treg population that exhibits the ideal biological features of a Treg therapeutic while the highly suppressive memory Tregs should be purposefully excluded from a Treg therapeutic due to their low lineage delity, low proliferative capacity, and greater pro-inflammatory potential [159]. Recently published results from The ONE study demonstrates that regulatory cell therapy is achievable and safe in living-donor kidney transplant recipients, and is associated with fewer infectious complications, but similar rejection rates in the first year. Therefore, immune cell therapy is a potentially useful therapeutic approach in recipients of kidney transplant to minimize the burden of general immunosuppression [160].

Finally, the immune capacity of the liver depends on the local hepatic and immune cells that transitory populate it. The current research provides abundant data about the intercellular tolerogenic mechanisms. However, some points need to be better clarified from the scientific and medical point of view. Among them are the fine-tuning of common immunosuppressive therapeutics regarding regulatory T cells, biochemical mechanisms of interactions between hepatocytes and immune cells, whether immune parameters of activation/suppression might provide information in advance about the liver function, the impact of individual immunogenetic variations on the recovery and operational tolerance etc. We think that the immune system should be considered as important player in the liver tolerance network and involved in the post-transplantation period monitoring.

8. Conclusion

The liver is a unique structure, where immunological mechanisms meet metabolic processes. The tightly regulated collaboration between them creates particular tolerogenic milieu that impacts the homeostatic state. Regulatory T cells are shown to play important role in these events. Their dynamic and function are promising for the further development of new biomarkers and treatment strategies in liver transplantation.

Acknowledgements

The authors are grateful to Sofia University, research grant No 10-122/24.04.2018.

Conflict of interest

The authors declare no conflict of interest.

Author details

Velislava Terzieva*, Yordanka Uzunova, Radosvet Gornev and Lubomir Spassov
Sofia University "Sveti Kliment Ohridski", Faculty of Medicine, Lozenets Hospital, Sofia, Bulgaria

*Address all correspondence to: velislava_terzieva@yahoo.com

IntechOpen

© 2020 The Author(s). Licensee IntechOpen. This chapter is distributed under the terms of the Creative Commons Attribution License (http://creativecommons.org/licenses/by/3.0), which permits unrestricted use, distribution, and reproduction in any medium, provided the original work is properly cited.

References

[1] Pons J et al. FoxP3 in Peripheral Blood Is Associated With Operational Tolerance in Liver Transplant Patients During Immunosuppression Withdrawal. Transplantation 2008 ; 86(10): 1370-8.

[2] Baroja-Mazo A et al. Tolerance in liver transplantation: Biomarkers and clinical relevance. World J Gastroenterology 2016; 22(34): 7676-91.

[3] Mederacke Y et al. Transient increase of activated regulatory T cells early after kidney transplantation. Sci Rep 2019; 9 (1021): 1-12.

[4] European Association for the Study of the Liver. EASL Clinical Practice Guidelines: Liver transplantation. J Hepatol 2016; 64(2): 433-85.

[5] Tanaka K ey al. Living donor liver transplantation: Eastern experiences. HPB 2004; 6(2): 88-94.

[6] Pashev V. Criteria for evaluating applicants for living donors in children's liver transplantation. Sofia University "Sveti Kliment Ohridski"; 2017.

[7] Uzunova Y. Liver transplantation in children (in Bulgarian). First Ed. Sofia: Professor Marin Drinov Publishing house of BAS; 2018.

[8] Yamamoto S et al. Liver Transplantation for Familial Amyloidotic Polyneuropathy (FAP): A Single-Center Experience Over 16 Years. Am J Transplant 2007; 7: 2597-604.

[9] Rela M et al. Auxiliary Partial Orthotopic Liver Transplantation for Crigler-Najjar Syndrome Type I. Ann Surgery 2. 1999; 29(4): 565-9.

[10] Moon J et al. Safety of small for size grafts in adult-to-adult living donor liver transplantation using the right lobe. Liver Transplantation 2010; 16: 864-869.

[11] Freitas-Lopes M et al. Differential Location and Distribution of Hepatic Immune Cells. Cells. 2017; 6(4): 48.

[12] Steinhoff *G. major* histocompatibility complex antigens in human liver transplants. J Hepatology 1990; 11(1): 9-15.

[13] Takeuchi O, Akira S. Pattern Recognition Receptors and Inflammation. Cell. 2010; 140: 805-20.

[14] Limmer A et al. Efficient presentation of exogenous antigen by liver endothelial cells to CD8+ T cells results in antigen-specific T-cell tolerance. Nat Med. 2000; 6(12): 1348-54.

[15] Diehl L et al. Tolerogenic maturation of liver sinusoidal endothelial cells promotes B7-homolog 1-dependent CD8+ T cell tolerance. Hepatology. 2008; 47(1): 296-305.

[16] Tilg H, Moschen A. Evolution of inflammation in nonalcoholic fatty liver disease: The multiple parallel hits hypothesis. Hepatology. 2010; 52(5): 1836-46.

[17] Filipe A, McLauchlan J. Hepatitis C virus and lipid droplets: Finding a niche. Trends in Molecular Medicine. 2015; 21(1): 34-42.

[18] Bar-Yishay I, Shaul Y, Shlomai A. Hepatocyte metabolic signalling pathways and regulation of hepatitis B virus expression. Liver International. 2011; 31: 282-90.

[19] O'Neill L, Pearce E. Immunometabolism governs dendritic cell and macrophage function. J Exp Med. 2016; 213(1): 15-23.

[20] Shi J et al. Cytokines and Abnormal Glucose and Lipid Metabolism. Front Endocrinol (Lausanne). 2019; 10: 1-16.

[21] Wilson G, Tennant D, McKeating J. Hypoxia inducible factors in liver disease and hepatocellular carcinoma: current understanding and future directions. J Hepatol. 2914; 61: 1397-406.

[22] Dinarello C. Therapeutic strategies to reduce IL-1 activity in treating local and systemic inflammation. Current Opinion in Pharmacology. 2004; 4: 378-85.

[23] Tsutsui H, Cai X, Hayashi S. Interleukin-1 Family Cytokines in Liver Diseases. Mediators Inflamm. 2015; 2015: 630265.

[24] Ren K, Torres R. Role of interleukin-1β during pain and inflammation. Brain Res Rev. 2009; 60(1): 57-64.

[25] Korkmaz B et al. Neutrophil elastase, proteinase 3, and cathepsin G as therapeutic targets in human diseases. Pharmacological Reviews. 2010; 62: 726-59.

[26] Coeshott C et al. Converting enzyme-independent release of tumor necrosis factor α and IL-1β from a stimulated human monocytic cell line in the presence of activated neutrophils or purified proteinase 3. Proc Natl Acad Sci U S A. 1999; 96(11): 6261-6.

[27] Meyer-Hoffert U, Wiedow O. Neutrophil serine proteases: Mediators of innate immune responses. Curr Opin Hematol. 2011; 18(1): 19-24.

[28] Blander J. A long-awaited merger of the pathways mediating host defence and programmed cell death. Vol. 14, Nature Reviews Immunology. 2014; 14: 601-18.

[29] Mirea AM et al. IL-1 Family Cytokine Pathways Underlying NAFLD: Towards New Treatment Strategies. Trends Mol Med. 2018; 24(5): 458-71.

[30] Racanelli V. The liver as an immunological organ. Hepatology. 2006; 43: 54-62.

[31] Kubes P, Jenne C. Immune Responses in the Liver. Annu Rev Immunol. 2018; 36: 247-77.

[32] Jiang Y et al. The Role of Diverse Liver Cells in Liver Transplantation Tolerance. Front Immunol. 2020; 11:1-16.

[33] Wiegard C et al. Defective T Helper Response of Hepatocyte-Stimulated CD4 T Cells Impairs Antiviral CD8 Response and Viral Clearance. Gastroenterology. 2007; 133(6): 2010-8.

[34] Herkel J et al. MHC class II-expressing hepatocytes function as antigen-presenting cells and activate specific CD4 T lymphocytes. Hepatology. 2003; 37(5): 1079-85.

[35] DeTemple D et al. Hepatocyte-induced CD4+ T cell alloresponse is associated with major histocompatibility complex class II up-regulation on hepatocytes and suppressible by regulatory T cells. Liver Transplantation. 2018; 24(3): 407-19.

[36] Burghardt S et al. Hepatocytes induce Foxp3 + regulatory T cells by Notch signaling . J Leukoc Biol. 2014; 96(4): 571-7.

[37] Kawai T, Akira S. The role of pattern-recognition receptors in innate immunity: Update on toll-like receptors. Vol. 11, Nature Immunology. 2010; 11: 373-84.

[38] You Q et al. Mechanism of T cell tolerance induction by murine hepatic Kupffer cells. Hepatology. 2008; 48(3): 978-90.

[39] Sørensen K et al. Liver sinusoidal endothelial cells. Compr Physiol. 2015; 5(4): 1751-74.

[40] Bilzer M, Roggel F, Gerbes A. Role of Kupffer cells in host defense and liver disease. Liver International. 2006; 26: 1175-86.

[41] Li P et al. The role of Kupffer cells in hepatic diseases. Vol. 85, Molecular Immunology. 2017; 85: 222-9.

[42] Xie Z et al. Intrahepatic PD-1/PD-L1 Up-regulation Closely Correlates with Inflammation and Virus Replication in Patients with Chronic HBV Infection. Immunol Invest. 2009; 38(7): 624-38.

[43] Gugenheim J et al. Specific absorption of lymphocytotoxic alloantibodies by the liver in inbred rats. Transplantation. 1990; 50(2): 309-13.

[44] Knoll P et al. Human Kupffer cells secrete IL-10 in response to lipopolysaccharide (LPS) challenge. J Hepatol. 1995; 22(2): 226-9.

[45] Morita M et al. Rejection triggers liver transplant tolerance: Involvement of mesenchyme-mediated immune control mechanisms in mice. Hepatology. 2015; 62(3): 915-31.

[46] Reynaert H et al. Hepatic stellate cells: Role in microcirculation and pathophysiology of portal hypertension. Gut. 2002; 50(4): 571-81.

[47] Wake K. "Sternzellen" in the liver: Perisinusoidal cells with special reference to storage of vitamin A. Am J Anat. 1971; 132(4): 429-62.

[48] Tsuchida T, Friedman S. Mechanisms of hepatic stellate cell activation. Nat Rev Gastroenterol Hepatol. 2017; 14(7): 397-411.

[49] Charles R et al. Human hepatic stellate cells inhibit t-cell response through B7-H1 pathway. Transplantation. 2013; 96(1): 17-24

[50] Mühlbauer M et al. PD-L1 is induced in hepatocytes by viral infection and by interferon-α and -γ and mediates T cell apoptosis. J Hepatol. 2006; 45(4): 520-8.

[51] Feldstein A et al. Hepatocyte apoptosis and Fas expression are prominent features of human nonalcoholic steatohepatitis. Gastroenterol. 2003; 125(2): 437-43.

[52] Höchst B et al. Activated human hepatic stellate cells induce myeloid derived suppressor cells from peripheral blood monocytes in a CD44-dependent fashion. J Hepatol. 2013; 59(3): 528-35.

[53] Kelly A et al. CD141+ myeloid dendritic cells are enriched in healthy human liver. J Hepatol. 2014; 60(1): 135-42.

[54] Steptoe R et al. Augmentation of Dendritic Cells in Murine Organ Donors by Flt3 Ligand Alters the Balance between Transplant Tolerance and Immunity. J Immunol. 1997; 159(11): 5483-91.

[55] Soysa R, Wu X, Crispe I. Dendritic cells in hepatitis and liver transplantation. Liver Transplantation. 2017; 23(11): 1433-9.

[56] Yokota S et al. Liver transplantation in the mouse: Insights into liver immunobiology, tissue injury, and allograft tolerance. Liver Transplantation. 2016; 22: 536-46.

[57] Bamboat Z et al. Human Liver Dendritic Cells Promote T Cell Hyporesponsiveness. J Immunol. 2009; 182(4): 1901-11.

[58] Thomson A, Knolle P. Antigen-presenting cell function in the tolerogenic liver environment. Nature Reviews Immunology. 2010; 10: 753-66.

[59] Raïch-Regué D, Glancy M, Thomson A. Regulatory dendritic cell therapy: From rodents to clinical application. Immunology Letters. 2014; 161: 216-21.

[60] Castellaneta A et al. NOD2 Ligation Subverts IFN-α Production by Liver Plasmacytoid Dendritic Cells and Inhibits Their T Cell Allostimulatory Activity via B7-H1 Up-Regulation. J Immunol. 2009; 183(11): 6922-32.

[61] Ibrahim J et al. Dendritic cell populations with different concentrations of lipid regulate tolerance and immunity in mouse and human liver. Gastroenterology. 2012; 143(4): 1061-72.

[62] Pillarisetty V et al. Liver Dendritic Cells Are Less Immunogenic Than Spleen Dendritic Cells because of Differences in Subtype Composition. J Immunol. 2004; 172(2): 1009-17.

[63] Klugewitz K et al. The composition of intrahepatic lymphocytes: Shaped by selective recruitment? Trends Immunol. 2004; 25(11): 590-4.

[64] Peng H, Tian Z. Re-examining the origin and function of liver-resident NK cells. Trends in Immunology. 2015; 36(5): 293-9.

[65] Heymann F, Tacke F. Immunology in the liver-from homeostasis to disease. Nat Rev Gastroenterol Hepatol. 2016; 13(2): 88-110.

[66] Tang X et al. IL-7 Licenses Activation of Human Liver Intrasinusoidal Mucosal-Associated Invariant T Cells. J Immunol. 2013; 190(7): 3142-52.

[67] Slichter C et al. Distinct activation thresholds of human conventional and innate-like memory T cells. JCI Insight. 2016; 1(8): e86292.

[68] Fontenot J, Gavin M, Rudensky A. Foxp3 programs the development and function of CD4+CD25+ regulatory T cells. Nat Immunol. 2003; 4: 330-6.

[69] Sakaguchi S. et al. Immunologic Self-Tolerance Maintained by Activated T Cells Expressing11-2 Receptor a-Chains (CD25). J Immunol. 1995; 155: 1151-64.

[70] Abbas A et al. Regulatory T cells : recommendations to simplify the nomenclature. Nat Publ Gr. 2013; 14(4): 307-8.

[71] Haas J et al. Prevalence of Newly Generated Naive Regulatory T Cells (T reg) Is Critical for T reg Suppressive Function and Determines T reg Dysfunction in Multiple Sclerosis. J Immunol. 2007; 179(2): 1322-30.

[72] Ahern D, Lloyd C, Robinson D. Chemokine responsiveness of CD4+ CD25+ regulatory and CD4+ CD25- T cells from atopic and nonatopic donors. Allergy Eur J Allergy Clin Immunol. 2009; 64(8): 1121-9.

[73] Kleinewietfeld M et al. CCR6 expression defines regulatory effector/memory-like cells within the CD25+CD4+ T-cell subset. Blood. 2005; 105(7): 2877-86.

[74] Zheng Y et al. Role of conserved non-coding DNA elements in the Foxp3 gene in regulatory T-cell fate. Nature. 2010; 463(1476-4687): 808-12.

[75] Lee W, Lee G. Transcriptional regulation and development of regulatory T cells. Exp Mol Med. 2018; 50(3): e456.

[76] Ohkura N, Kitagawa Y, Sakaguchi S. Development and maintenance of regulatory T cells. Immunity. 2013; 38: 414-23.

[77] Heltemes-harris L et al. The role of STAT5 in the development, function,

and transformation of B and T lymphocytes. Ann N Y Acad Sci. 2011; 1217: 18-31.

[78] Lio C, Hsieh C. A Two-Step Process for Thymic Regulatory T Cell Development. Immunity. 2008; 28(1):1 00-11.

[79] Burchill M et al. Linked T Cell Receptor and Cytokine Signaling Govern the Development of the Regulatory T Cell Repertoire. Immunity. 2008; 28(1): 112-21.

[80] Goldstein J et al. Inhibition of the JAK/STAT signaling pathway in regulatory T cells reveals a very dynamic regulation of foxp3 expression. PLoS One. 2016; 11(4) :1-16.

[81] Cao R et al. Role of Histone H3 Lysine 27 Methylation in Polycomb-Group Silencing. Science. 2002; 298(5595): 1039-43.

[82] Arvey A et al. Inflammation-induced repression of chromatin bound by the transcription factor Foxp3 in regulatory T cells. Nat imonol. 2014; 15(6): 580-587.

[83] Yang X et al. EZH2 is crucial for both differentiation of regulatory T cells and T effector cell expansion. Sci Rep. 2015; 5(1): 10643.

[84] Mabarrack N, Turner N, Mayrhofer G. Recent thymic origin, differentiation, and turnover of regulatory T cells. J Leukoc Biol. 2008; 84(5): 1287-97.

[85] Bettini M, Vignali D. Development of Thymically-Derived Natural Regulatory T Cells. Ann N Y Acad Sci. 2010; 3(1183): 1-12.

[86] Marcovecchio G et al. Thymic Epithelium Abnormalities in DiGeorge and Down Syndrome Patients Contribute to Dysregulation in T Cell Development. Front Immunol. 2019; 10:1-15.

[87] Josefowicz S, Lu L, Rudensky A. Regulatory T Cells: Mechanisms of Differentiation and Function. Annu Rev Immunol. 2012; 30: 531-64.

[88] Cowan J, Jenkinson W, Anderson G. Thymus medulla fosters generation of natural Treg cells, invariant γδ T cells, and invariant NKT cells: What we learn from intrathymic migration. Eur J Immunol. 2015; 45(3): 652-60.

[89] Tuovinen H et al. The FOXP3+subset of human CD4+CD8+thymocytes is immature and subject to intrathymic selection. Immunol Cell Biol. 2008; 86(6): 523-9.

[90] Lan Q et al. Induced Foxp3 + regulatory T cells: A potential new weapon to treat autoimmune and inflammatory diseases? J Mol Cell Biol. 2012; 4(1): 22-8.

[91] Lee J et al. Progesterone Promotes Differentiation of Human Cord Blood Fetal T Cells into T Regulatory Cells but Suppresses Their Differentiation into Th17 Cells. J Immunol. 2011; 187(4): 1778-87.

[92] Piccioni M et al. T Helper Cell Differentiation and Their Function. 2014; 841 : 67-97.

[93] Takahashi T. et al. Immunologic self-tolerance maintained by CD25(+) CD4(+) regulatory T cells constitutively expressing cytotoxic T lymphocyte-associated antigen 4. J Exp Med. 2000; 192(2): 303-10.

[94] Dilek N et al. Targeting CD28, CTLA-4 and PD-L1 costimulation differentially controls immune synapses and function of human regulatory and conventional t-cells. PLoS One. 2013; 8(12): 2-15.

[95] Terness P et al. Inhibition of allogeneic T cell proliferation by indoleamine 2,3-dioxygenase-expressing dendritic cells: Mediation of suppression by tryptophan metabolites. J Exp Med. 2002; 196(4): 447-57.

[96] Gotot J et al. Regulatory T cells use programmed death 1 ligands to directly suppress autoreactive B cells in vivo. Proc Natl Acad Sci U S A. 2012; 109(26): 10468-73.

[97] Ghebeh H ey al. FOXP3+ Tregs and B7-H1+/PD-1+ T lymphocytes co-infiltrate the tumor tissues of high-risk breast cancer patients: Implication for immunotherapy. BMC Cancer. 2008; 8: 57.

[98] Fife B et al. Interactions between PD-1 and PD-L1 promote tolerance by blocking the TCR-induced stop signal. Nat Immunol. 2009; 10(11): 1185-92.

[99] Franceschini D et al. PD-L1 negatively regulates CD4+CD25+Foxp3+ Tregs by limiting STAT-5 phosphorylation in patients chronically infected with HCV. J Clin Invest. 2009; 119(3): 551-64.

[100] Bacchetta R et al. Growth and expansion of human T regulatory type 1 cells are independent from TCR activation but require exogenous cytokines. Eur J Immunol. 2002; 32(8): 2237-45.

[101] Cosmi L et al. Human CD8+CD25+ thymocytes share phenotypic and functional features with CD4+CD25+ regulatory thymocytes. Blood. 2003; 102(12): 4107-14.

[102] Bézie S et al. IL-34 is a Treg-specific cytokine and mediates transplant tolerance. J Clin Invest. 2015; 125(10): 3952-64.

[103] Collison L et al. Interleukin-35-mediated induction of a novel regulatory T cell population. Nat Immunol. 2011; 11(12): 1093-101.

[104] Sawant D V., Hamilton K, Vignali DAA. Interleukin-35: Expanding Its Job Profile. J Interf Cytokine Res [Internet]. 2015;35(7):499-512.

[105] Grossman W et al. Human T regulatory cells can use the perforin pathway to cause autologous target cell death. Immun. 2004; 21: 589-601.

[106] Valencia X et al. TNF downmodulates the function of human CD4+CD25hiT-regulatory cells. Blood. 2006; 108(1): 253-61.

[107] Chen X et al. TNFR2 Is Critical for the Stabilization of the CD4+Foxp3+ Regulatory T Cell Phenotype in the Inflammatory Environment. J Immunol. 2013; 190(3): 1076-84.

[108] Chen X, Oppenheim J. TNF-α : An Activator of CD4 + FoxP3 + TNFR2 + Regulatory T Cells. TNF Pathophysiol Mol Cell Mech. 2010; 11: 119-34.

[109] Caudy A et al. CD25 deficiency causes an immune dysregulation, polyendocrinopathy, enteropathy, X-linked-like syndrome, and defective IL-10expression from CD4 lymphocytes. J Allergy Clin Immunol. 2007; (119): 482-487.

[110] Goudy K et al. Human IL2RA null mutation mediates immunodeficiency with lymphoproliferation and autoimmunity. Clin Immunol. 2013; 146(3): 248-61.

[111] Ferreira R et al. Cells with Treg-specific FOXP3 demethylation but low CD25 are prevalent in autoimmunity. J Autoimmun. 2017; 84: 75-86.

[112] Barron L et al. Cutting edge: mechanisms of IL-2- dependent maintenance of functional regulatory T cells. J Immunol. 2010; 185: 6426-30.

[113] Cheng G, Yu A, Malek T. T-cell tolerance and the multi-functional role of IL-2R signaling in Tregulatory cells. Immunol Rev. 2011; 241(1): 63-76.

[114] Demetris A, Isse K. Tissue biopsy monitoring of operational tolerance in liver allograft recipients.Current Opinion in Organ Transplantation. 2013; 18: 345-53.

[115] Ashton-Chess J et al. Spontaneous operational tolerance after immunosuppressive drug withdrawal in clinical renal allotransplantation. Vol. 84, Transplantation. 2007; 84: 1215-9.

[116] Di Cocco P et al. Clinical Operational Tolerance After Solid Organ Transplantation. Transplant Proc. 2009; 41(4): 1278-82.

[117] Orlando G, Soker S, Wood K. Operational tolerance after liver transplantation. J Hepatol. 2009; 50(6): 1247-57.

[118] Li Y et al. Analyses of peripheral blood mononuclear cells in operational tolerance after pediatric living donor liver transplantation. Am J Transplant. 2004; 4(12): 2118-25.

[119] Koshiba T et al. Clinical, immunological, and pathological aspects of operational tolerance after pediatric living-donor liver transplantation. Transpl Immunol. 2007; 17(2): 94-7.

[120] Demirkiran A et al. Low circulating regulatory T-cell levels after acute rejection in liver transplantation. Liver Transplant. 2006; 12(2): 277-84.

[121] Demirkiran A et al. Allosuppressive Donor CD4 + CD25 + Regulatory T Cells Detach from the Graft and Circulate in Recipients after Liver Transplantation . J Immunol. 2007; 178(10): 6066-72.

[122] Terzieva V et al. The Dynamic Changes in Soluble CD30 and Regulatory T Cells Before and After Solid Organ Transplantations: A Pilot Study. Monoclon Antib Immunodiagn Immunother. 2019; 38(4): 137-44.

[123] Baumann A et al. Preferential accumulation of T helper cells but not cytotoxic T cells characterizes benign subclinical rejection of human liver allografts. Liver Transplant. 2016; 22(7): 943-55.

[124] Billingham R, Brent L, Medawar P. "Actively acquired tolerance" of foreign cells. Nature. 1953; 172(4379): 603-6.

[125] Jonsson J et al. Peripheral blood chimerism following human liver transplantation. Hepatology. 1997; 25(5): 1233-6.

[126] Wu S, Pan C. Tolerance and chimerism and allogeneic bone marrow/stem cell transplantation in liver transplantation. World J Gastroenterol. 2013; 19(36): 5981-7.

[127] Abrol N, Jadlowiec C, Taner T. Revisiting liver's role in transplant alloimmunity. World J Gastroenterol. 2019; 25(25): 3123-35.

[128] Takatsuki M et al. Analysis of alloreactivity and intragraft cytokine profiles in living donor liver transplant recipients with graft acceptance. Transpl Immunol. 2001; 8(4): 279-86.

[129] Martinez-Llordella M et al. Multiparameter immune profiling of operational tolerance in liver transplantation. Am J Transplant. 2007; 7(2): 309-19.

[130] Wiendl H. Fast track to becoming a regulatory T cell : " trogocytosis " of HLA-G. 2014; 109(5): 1796-7.

[131] Lozano J et al. CD8 + HLA-G + Regulatory T Cells Are Expanded in HIV-1-Infected Patients . Viral Immunol. 2009; 22(6): 463-5.

[132] Castellaneta A et al. HLA-G level on monocytoid dendritic cells correlates with regulatory T-cell Foxp3 expression in liver transplant tolerance. Transplantation. 2011; 91(10): 1132-40.

[133] LeMaoult J et al. Immune regulation by pretenders: Cell-to-cell transfers of HLA-G make effector T cells act as regulatory cells. Blood. 2007; 109(5): 2040-48.

[134] Lila N et al. Human leukocyte antigen-G expression after heart transplantation is associated with a reduced incidence of rejection. Circulation. 2002; 105(16): 1949-54.

[135] Luque J et al. Soluble HLA-G in Heart Transplantation: Their Relationship to Rejection Episodes and Immunosuppressive Therapy. Hum Immunol. 2006; 67(4-5): 257-63.

[136] Terasaki P. Tolerogenic Mechanisms in Liver Transplantation. SOJ Immunol. 2015; 3(4): 01-13.

[137] Amiot L, Vu N, Samson M. Biology of the immunomodulatory molecule HLA-G in human liver diseases. J Hepatol. 2015; 62(6): 1430-7.

[138] González-Hernandez A et al. Linking two immuno-suppressive molecules: Indoleamine 2,3 dioxygenase can modify HLA-G cell-surface expression. Biol Reprod. 2005; 73(3): 571-8.

[139] Fukusato T et al. Expression of HLA class I antigens on hepatocytes in liver disease. Am J Pathol 1986;123: 264-270.

[140] Zarkhin V et al. Expression of soluble HLA-G identifies favorable outcomes in liver transplant recipients. Transplantation. 2010; 90(9): 1000-5.

[141] Crispim J et al. Human leukocyte antigen-G expression after kidney transplantation is associated with a reduced incidence of rejection. Transpl Immunol. 2008; 18(4): 361-7.

[142] Waid D et al. Defining a new biomarker for the autoimmune component of Multiple Sclerosis: Th40 cells. J Neuroimmunol. 2014; 270(1-2): 75-85.

[143] Tselios K et al. CD4+CD25highFOXP3+ T regulatory cells as a biomarker of disease activity in systemic lupus erythematosus: A prospective study. Clin Exp Rheumatol. 2014; 32(5): 630-9.

[144] Baraka A, Salem H. Clinical significance of T-regulatory cells in B-cell non-Hodgkin's lymphoma. Egypt J Immunol. 2011; 18(2): 23-30.

[145] Jagasia M et al. KD025-208: A Phase 2a Study of KD025 for Patients with Chronic Graft Versus Host Disease (cGVHD) — Pharmacodynamics and Updated Results. Blood. 2018; 132(Supplement 1): 602.

[146] Abdolmohammadi-Vahid S et al. Intravenous immunoglobulin (IVIG) modulates regulatory T cells and improves pregnancy outcome in patients with repeated implantation failure (RIF). Syst Biol Reprod Med. 2017; 63(6): 350-9.

[147] Robertson S, Care A, Moldenhauer L. Regulatory T cells in embryo implantation and the immune response to pregnancy. J Clin Invest. 2018; 128(10): 4224-35.

[148] Barzaghi F, Passerini L, Bacchetta R. Immune dysregulation, polyendocrinopathy, enteropathy, X-linked syndrome: A paradigm of immunodeficiency with autoimmunity. Front Immunol. 2012; 3: 1-25.

[149] Janson P et al. FOXP3 promoter demethylation reveals the committed Treg population in humans. PLoS One. 2008; 3(2): e1612.

[150] Angerami M et al. Expansion of CD25-negative forkhead Box P3-positive T cells during HIV and *Mycobacterium tuberculosis* infection. Front Immunol. 2017; 8: 1-12.

[151] Brunet M et al. Barcelona Consensus on Biomarker-Based Immunosuppressive Drugs Management in Solid Organ Transplantation. Ther Drug Monit. 2016; 38(Suppl 1): 1-20.

[152] Heidt S, Wood K. Biomarkers of operational tolerance in solid organ transplantation. Expert Opin Med Diagn. 2012; 6(4): 281-93.

[153] Xiao F et al. Ex vivo expanded human regulatory T cells delay islet allograft rejection via inhibiting islet-derived monocyte chemoattractant protein-1 production in CD34+ stem cells-reconstituted NOD-scid IL2rγnull mice. PLoS One. 2014; 9(3): e90387.

[154] Xia G, He J, Leventhal J. Ex vivo-expanded natural CD4+CD25+ regulatory T cells synergize with host T-cell depletion to promote long-term survival of allografts. Am J Transplant. 2008; 8(2): 298-306.

[155] Meijer B, Rutten V, Aijtink V, Scalera I, Mihaylov V, Heikkila K, Pegel L, Perera T, Hartog H. Safety of intraoperative blood salvage during liver transplantation in patients with hepatocellular carcinoma ; systemic review and meta-analysis. Transplant International 2017, vol.30 (Suppl.2), 8-164 (94).

[156] Johnston L et al. A Phase I Study of Donor Regulatory T Cells As Treatment for Steroid Dependent/Refractory Chronic Graft Versus Host Disease. Blood. 2016; 128(22): 385-385.

[157] Haarer J et al. Early Enrichment and Restitution of the Peripheral Blood Treg Pool Is Associated With Rejection-Free Stable Immunosuppression After Liver Transplantation. Transplantation. 2016; 100(7): e39-40.

[158] Todo S et al. A pilot study of operational tolerance with a regulatory T-cell-based cell therapy in living donor liver transplantation. Hepatology. 2016; 64(2): 632-643.

[159] Donnelly C et al. Optimizing human Treg immunotherapy by Treg subset selection and E-selectin ligand expression. Sci Rep. 2018; 8(1): 1-14.

[160] Sawitzki B et al. Regulatory cell therapy in kidney transplantation (The ONE Study): a harmonised design and analysis of seven non-randomised, single-arm, phase 1/2A trials. Lancet. 2020; 395(10237): 1627-39.

Section 4

New Frontiers in Organ Transplantation

Chapter 7

Coupling and Deviating of Altruism-Voluntariness Relationship in Organ Transplantation

Mesut Güvenbaş and Omur Sayligil

Abstract

Organ transplantation is an issue that concerns two people (donor and recipient) at the same time in terms of the right to life, which is the most basic human right. The direct utility arising from organ transplantation involves the patient to whom the organ is transplanted, and the indirect utility relates to the donor. Today, the decision to obtain an organ from a living donor is based on the idea of doing something good by those who sacrifice themselves for their relatives. The person who donates an organ treats their body as an instrument and uses their willpower on it. If the statement "I will care about the health of others" is accepted as a universal principle, it will be very important to establish a balance between the duty of caring for the health of others and protecting one's own health. If we want to introduce a new approach to be adopted in the assessment of living donors in society, we must look at the real situation in terms of utility, altruism, and volunteering. This Chapter thus evaluates organ transplantation from living donors in terms of utility, altruism, and volunteering.

Keywords: altruism, voluntariness, organ transplantation, autonomy, pre-transplantation assessment

1. Introduction

Wouldn't the world be a better place if there were no limits to sacrifice? Most people will answer yes to this question. When it comes to organ transplantation, can this fact occasionally contradict primum non nocere, "first, do no harm", which is the basic doctrine of medicine. Although selfishness is rarely accepted as a strategy for the benefit of the group, in evolutionary formulation, altruism benefits the group and selfishness interferes with altruism. While the living donor benefits the person who needs organ transplantation, they assume a group of life risks in advance. In this case, assessments will be multi-layered. Can the recipient's physician take a paternalistic approach to the benefit of their patient? How much risk can the donor take with the thought of benefiting another person? How should the decision of the potential donor to donate organs be handled? How should the organ donation decision based on their altruistic approach be evaluated within the scope of autonomy? Do the risks undertaken by the donor mean that they will be harmed?

It is of course possible to augment the number of questions, but the need for organ transplantation is increasing every other day. The number of donors does not match the needs, and this increases the need for organs every other day and causes the waiting lists for organs to get longer. Due to the scarcity of cadaver donations especially in some countries, organ transplantation, including kidney transplantation, is performed mainly from living donors.

With the increasing need for organs, organ transplantation from living donors, who are relatives of the recipient or not, is becoming more common, and even scientific studies on organ and tissue transplantation present living organ donors as an alternative to long-term dialysis treatment [1].

In justification of transplantation procedures with organs obtained from living donors, one has to be genuinely volunteer and to give informed consent under free will. Saving an individual's life and donating living organs can be a commendable option. However, to make sure the utility reaches its aim, a balance must be maintained between the utility provided to the sick person and the cost that the person taking an altruistic approach will pay. It should be essential to minimize the damage and maximize the possible utility in organ transplantation practice.

Various ethical statements suggest that the individual should voluntarily donate organs of their free will by giving informed consent, the donation should be exempt from exploitation and pressure, the donor should have the freedom to withdraw from the donation process at any time, and that the transplant team should make sure that the donor's decision to donate is voluntary and not manipulated. The correct definition of volunteering is an issue of practical importance. The answer to the question of how donors' volunteering should be properly assessed is far from a resolution today. Although standards about informing donors and how to control the information they understand have been developed (for example, the US Medicare Program), an empirical assessment standard of whether the decision to donate is voluntary is not developed enough to meet the relevant ethical norms [2]. One of the most important studies on the topic is the one carried out by Al-Khader. This study aimed to develop a scoring and rating system for assessing the volunteering of potential living donors [3]. In light of, a scoring and grading model was proposed in our country too, to determine the volunteering of living donors in kidney transplantation [1].

The assessment of potential donors' willingness to volunteer for organ donation, which is basically a difficult process, handles issues, such as motivation to donate, social status and family ties, economic status, relationship with the recipient, evidence of volunteering, and proof of a financial reward. Various ethical guidelines on organ transplantation from living donors have been developed around the world. One of the first ethical guidelines suggested is "Consensus Statement on the Live Organ Donor" [4]. In the light of this guideline, other ethical guidelines for the assessment of living donors have been developed [5].

When living donors want to donate organs, it is important to determine whether they are really volunteers or whether they are subject to a relationship of interest or control over their volunteering. It is an ethical and legal requirement for the donor to donate of their free will and by fully volunteering. The creation of a measurement tool on organ transplant volunteering is considered to be important in terms of the value and non-instrumentalization of human beings.

Contrary to the expectations of transplant surgeons, the use of living donors in countries, such as Turkey, Saudi Arabia, or South Korea is increasing every other day, resulting in more transplants from living donors than cadavers [6].

Nowadays, with the acceptance of cross organ transplants and living organ donations from non-relatives, the issue of volunteering and altruism of volunteers has become much more important. Lack of a standard approach to these issues is one of the biggest problem areas.

Utility of organ transplantation is available to the recipient under all circumstances. Health business is a utilitarian business. For this reason, utility fits the basic philosophy of healthcare very well. However, no matter how the individual's actions are conditioned to positive and beneficial results, negative and undesirable consequences may accompany these beneficial results as well. In the context of doing no harm, one of the main topics that need to be addressed is who or what is responsible for the damage, if any, and the other is assessment of the damage. Undoubtedly, balancing the benefit and harm is of particular importance for high-risk healthcare providers.

2. Utility

Morality requires that we do not only avoid harming people and regard them as autonomous but also contribute to the well-being of other people. This is expressed under the title of "utility". Apart from avoiding harming others, people should take positive steps to help other people. The utility can be examined under the "positive utility" heading, which refers to the action of the subject to provide some benefits to others, and utility, which requires the subject to establish a balance between benefits, risks, and costs to achieve the best overall results [7]. Regarding our subject, it is necessary to talk about the utility and saving duty for the specific (i.e. for certain people) rather than the general benefit.

General utility targets all persons regardless of special relationships. The utility specific to persons emerging as a result of moral relationships, contracts, and special ties usually applies to certain persons, such as our children, friends, parties to the contract, or patients. Although the idea that we have an obligation to all people is controversial, almost everyone agrees with the idea that we have an obligation to act for the benefit of the people with whom we have special relationships [7].

Beauchamp and Childress argues that the "duty to save" requires an obligation to provide a prima facie utility if all of the following conditions are met, even if close moral relationships based on specific agreements or family and friendship ties are excluded.

1. Person Y is at risk of serious loss or damage to his life, health, or other fundamental interests.

2. The action of person X (alone or in the relevant chain of actions) is necessary to prevent this loss or damage.

3. The action of person X (alone or in combination with other actions) will most likely prevent this loss or damage.

4. Person X will not put himself/herself at any critical risk, cost, or burden by performing this action.

5. The expected benefits for person Y outweigh the damage, cost, or burden that person X may face [7].

In the light of these evaluations of Beauchamp and Childress, the 4th condition constitutes the debate on whether living donors who have a special contract for organ transplantation or have family and friendship ties have an obligatory saving mission. If we do not consider a person's donation of a kidney as "a critical risk, cost, or burden", then we put potential living donors under obligatory duty to save.

Putting the living donor, who will only have moral gains, under the direct obligation of compulsory saving would be a point in contradiction with the concept of volunteering. Also, another issue to discuss is which of the individuals who meet these conditions and have a family, friend, or special contractual relationships with the recipient will fulfill this obligation first.

It should be noted that the obligation to save is at the core of why living organ donors mostly donate organs to their relatives (family, friends, relatives, etc.). Even if the conditions stated by Beauchamp & Childress are met, it is a matter of debate whether we have an obligation to save people we do not know, especially in terms of organ transplantation. The fact that people hesitate to donate living organs to patients they do not know can be shown as evidence of this matter. Expecting such a sacrifice from the whole society will not go beyond pursuing a high ideal.

Balancing the duties of providing utility and doing no harm with the principles of respect for autonomy and justice is accepted as essential [8]. This balance requires the determination of the capacity and autonomy of living organ donors and the careful examination of the stages that require their voluntary consent.

In this context, the volunteering of living donors who want to give a "new life" to their family, friend, or someone they do not know as a living organ donor should be determined well, and the special utility action of the person should be ethically assessed within the concept of obligation to save.

The majority of scientists studying living organ donation ethics have reached a consensus on the issue that giving a certain level of harm to competent volunteers to save another person's life requires that a valid consent for the donation is available, living organ donation provides a general positive balance of harm and benefit that cannot be achieved in a way that is less damaging to donors and recipients, and that the donation does not lead to significant and long-term morbidity or mortality of the donor.

Altruism, which is also a piece of modesty, is the ability of a person to prefer someone else's purposes and desires over their own purposes and desires. Altruism, which is the most important factor underlying the expression of volunteering, is one of the basic principles of organ transplantation.

3. Altruism

Although there are partial similarities in the assessment of potential organ donors, there are regional differences in how assessments are carried out. The criteria explaining who is allowed to donate and who will be disqualified as a donor also differ.

Family members who make an organ donation will benefit from a successful organ transplant operation to their loved ones, which can be effective in the risk and benefit discussion during the approval process. It may be necessary to limit the sacrifice allowed. For example, while we do not accept a living heart donor for obvious reasons, we know that most donors can live with a single kidney.

It is difficult to predict whether a particular organ donation is an altruistic act because while most recipients benefit from the transplant, the recipient may be in a worse condition if an organ is rejected or the operation fails. As an altruistic action/practice is judged by the outcome, it is difficult to pre-operationally determine whether any special donation proposal is acceptable. Altruism is one of the basic principles of organ transplantation. In organ transplantation;

1. altruistic action must be an action that leads to an outcome,

2. the action should be directly linked to the aim,

3. the action should aim at enhancing another person's well-being or quality of life,

4. if the person wants to take action for another person, the result of the action, whether it is bad or it generates negative consequences in the long run, will not decrease the altruistic nature of that action [9].

3.1 Definitions of altruism and altruism in the context of organ transplantation

Merriam-Webster dictionary defines altruism as unselfish respect and commitment to the well-being of others [10]. The Contemporary Turkish Dictionary of the Turkish Language Association defines the concept of altruism as "the state of being altruistic, selflessness". The synonyms of altruist and altruism are given as selfless and selflessness. According to the same dictionary, an altruist is a person who tries to be useful to someone else without pursuing any personal benefits [11].

The word altruism is derived from the word alter, which comes from Latin meaning "other". In the 1830s, Auguste Comte used this word as a general term to mean "care for others". While altruism often points out to sparing thought for another, people can self-sacrifice due to environmental pressure while taking an altruistic approach. While volunteering and personal preference come to the fore in altruism, it may be possible for the person to act as a donor even if they are not willing. If a person acts with completely altruistic motives, that is, if the self-seeking motives are completely absent, we can define this action as a "pure" state of altruism. We must be careful to distinguish purely altruistic behavior from self-sacrificing behavior: the former does not pursue personal gains, while the latter involves some loss. Altruism is the opposite of egoism. However, the person who transcends egoism can be altruistic. A person, not who takes action in a situation where their interests are not harmed at all, but who does what is necessary in a situation that touches their own interests or who can do what should be done and act fairly will be altruistic.

Sacrifice can be seen as a manifestation of individual autonomy. In this case, it is necessary to accept a certain risk in advance. It is unavoidable that the operation to be performed to remove the transplantable graft is risky even if the donor's health is excellent. The short-term mortality risk for living kidney donors is roughly the same as the risk taken by any patient under general anesthesia. People take risks in their daily lives, which are far greater than the risks often imposed by donor surgery, with little or no direct benefit to their health. The risk of damage from kidney donation is much less compared to the many risks we all face in daily life. Therefore, if both the donor and the recipient are informed about the risks of the surgery, the long-term outcomes of the donation, and the forecast of factors that may affect the success of the transplant, the living organ donation will not push the limits of an acceptable sacrifice.

Schopenhauer mentions denial of the will, silencing the ego, and transcending egoism, which are essential for the existence of freedom, justice, and love in the world and says that this can occur in two ways: by gaining knowledge of the suffering of others or by the person's own great suffering. Schopenhauer says that the vast majority of those who deny the will achieve it in the latter way; not only by the acquisition of knowledge but also by the experience of pain. According to Kant I, the fact that action or the will at the basis of the action is determined by the self-love of maxims makes that action unethical. Therefore, it would not be wrong to say that morality and freedom can only be achieved when the person who determines the actions does not have desires and tendencies [8].

If a social behavior decreases the appropriateness of the organism performing the behavior but increases the suitability of others, it is considered an altruistic behavior. Although the concept of altruism was first introduced within the discipline of sociology, today it is frequently used in fields, such as sociology, psychology, theology, and education. Definitions of altruism handled in different perspectives and different disciplines naturally vary, too. In almost all disciplines, altruism is not understood as showing helping behavior without an expectation of personal reward or benefit. Should altruism be understood as the individual's consideration of well-being of others as much as his/her own or as seeing the well-being of others above his/her own? If a person sees others' well-being over/before his/her own, he/she will be seen to be sacrificing for others without expecting a response. When altruistic behavior is shown with the expectation of gaining benefit from the person sacrificing, this situation may sometimes appear in the form of cooperation or showing off.

Since the altruism in question here is realized with the expectation of self-interest, this situation is based on mutual altruism, and it can be said that altruism is a kind of strategy that aims to gain respect in society. Gaining public reputation and the desire to benefit from the new opportunities that society offers to them can also support this type of behavior. The person who acts altruistically in the latter form of altruistic behavior, which is based on volunteering without any expectation of benefit, and where the motivation to live for others is dominant, does not seek reward, and deterrent effects do not influence him/her in any way. It should not be forgotten that in the domain between these two views regarding altruism, a spiritual gain to be obtained from the person who has sacrificed will be dominant. It is in this domain that one's moral gains in return for altruistic behavior are called theological and moral altruism [12].

The most important factor that distinguishes altruism from other purposive behaviors such as "helping" and "obeying social rules" is that the altruist sacrifices something from themselves and takes on a burden depending on their behaviors. This burden distinguishes altruistic behavior from individual behavior, such as "benevolent" or "kind, manners". The behavior of the altruist, which emerges in social life and is "for the benefit of someone else but brings harm to themselves", varies by the conditions, the cause that leads to the behavior, and the behavior process. For this reason, the concept of altruism also swings between Kropotkin's understanding of absolute altruism [13] and mutual altruism approaches based on expectations.

Pro-social behaviors include behaviors that may be for the benefit of another person or a group, which are shown without being under pressure and voluntarily. Bierhoff [14] distinguishes helping behavior, pro-social behavior, and altruistic behavior as follows. Helping is a broad term covering all types of interpersonal support. Pro-social behavior is a rather narrower concept than helping because the action is intended to improve the status of the recipient, and the recipient is not an institution but a person. Altruism, on the other hand, is pro-social behavior, which means that with an additional restriction, the motivation of the person who helps is determined by perspective acquisition and empathy.

The proportion of healthy adults who are potentially able to donate kidneys is greater than the number of deaths under conditions that comply with a donation. The number of people willing to donate instead is limited. It is not surprising that a healthy person may be reluctant to undergo surgery without clinical benefit, and some donors in most countries donate to family or close friends. Some factors affecting this situation, such as the number of people waiting for transplantation and the benefits of organ donation, can be presented through various channels, and this can highlight the person in terms of donation. Some organ donation campaigns have featured individual 'case studies', which are sometimes called 'stories of hope' that tell the story of people awaiting a transplant and describing their situation and highlight the benefits a transplant can provide. The use of case studies aims to motivate and address people to take action to help others and create empathy by making the human impact of organ deficiency clearer.

The empathic-altruism hypothesis, widely described and proven in the psychological literature, suggests that empathic anxiety for another can lead to altruistic motivation to improve the well-being of the other [15].

Traditionally, altruism refers to a situation where one takes action for the benefit of another even when self-sacrifice is required. Therefore, altruism shows up with actions since goodwill and good thoughts are alone not enough. One goal of this action should include helping another person. If the well-being of the other person is an unintentional or secondary result of an action that one takes to improve one's own well-being, this action is not altruistic. Altruism does not change according to circumstances. Considering these characteristics, altruistic people are those who have a feeling of caring/considering other people.

There is no widely accepted classification of the types of altruism; however, two types of altruism, normative and hedonistic, are mentioned in some studies. While **normative altruism** can emerge through moral intuition, non-moral social rules, or logic, **hedonistic altruism** emphasizes that the individual finds a value in their perception of the situation where other individuals' distress decreases, they are better off, or they are happier [16].

Ethical altruism is based on the principle that altruism is a virtue, even an obligation. Some might argue that people are always generous and altruistic. This view may apply to a sole advocate of ethical altruism. At this point, the person expressing opinion actually advocates **psychological altruism**. It is worth noting the consequences of **pure altruism**-related behaviors based on the fact that everyone accepts the assumption of desiring very little for themselves and very much for others by one's voluntary sacrifice of their own pleasure to give pleasure to others. All those who behave in this way should not have thoughts for themselves as the giver, nor for others as the recipient, when considered not only as the waiver but as the acceptor of what has been renounced. A sense of compassion that is worrisome for others, willingly self-victimizing to benefit others, cannot be achieved without thinking that those who victimize themselves by giving something to others expect a benefit from it [17].

Moral altruism is based on rewarding the altruistic and punishing those who are not altruistic [18].

Kin altruism is defined as the situation where an individual jeopardizes their own safety to increase the survival chance of other people with genetic or blood ties in the same family [19].

Generally, the living donor is an adult family member whose first-degree relative has terminal stage renal disease. Their experience provides them with insight into the challenges of kidney disease and transplantation. Individuals, motivated by altruism when they choose to donate kidneys after thinking for a long time about risks and benefits, can be emotionally unsettled, and even if they believe they are acting with a desire to help, their ability to act autonomously and without coercion may be endangered.

When the priority of the family concerning organ donation is considered in the blood tie theory, the emergence of altruistic behavior is explained by kin relationships. The individual behaves more altruistically towards their close relatives who carry the same genes, such as mother vs. child, and siblings vs. siblings, compared to other individuals. As the blood ties decrease, the desire to tolerate harm for altruistic behavior or the likelihood of the emergence of altruistic behavior decreases.

The reason for this is that human beings have gone through a psychological evolution process in a way that motivates them to spare even their lives in order for their own genes to be permanent. Thus, a person who has close relations to an altruistic individual can survive through the behavior of this altruistic relative.

Partial altruism, which means the individual shares their assets with others, also constitutes an example of altruism approaches, especially in organ transplantation. While doing a favor to others, the person may have sometimes thought of obtaining financial gains from this behavior.

Living donors without a genetic link are increasingly used worldwide, and various approaches support the application. Donors who are not genetically linked to the recipient and who are emotionally connected to the patient and motivated by a desire to help, without an expectation of any material gains can be examples of partial altruism. Many psychological studies show people behave more altruistically towards their friends who have strong emotional bonds with compared to others even though they have no kin relationship. In a meta-analysis investigating factors related to organ donation [20], it was found that education, religion, knowledge, attitude, social influence, altruism, and family positively affected organ donation and that fear of death and the fear of organ donation negatively impacted it.

Pro-social behavior has been suggested by some social scientists as the opposite of anti-social behavior and has been defined as a behavior done with autonomous and free will that benefits others. According to Batson, there are two types of pro-social behavior: egocentric and other-centered. In egocentric pro-social behavior, the person expects to be rewarded or escape from any negativity for the positive behavior to another, while in other-centered pro-social behavior, the only goal of the person is to be helpful to the person to whom the positive behavior is directed, and there is no personal expectation in return for this behavior [21]. While this type of behavior is specified as altruistic behavior, one of the best examples of this is organ donation after death. A person cannot benefit from donating their organs after death.

In a study on the phenomenon of altruistic behavior, titled "An investigation on epistemological problems", Yeşilkaya approaches the subject with a three-color classification. The view claiming that altruism is based on the expectation of gaining a benefit from the person or the community that receives the sacrifice is characterized by the "black" metaphor, and the view claiming that this kind of sacrifice is made without expecting any return from any source is characterized by the "white" metaphor. However, when the research on this subject is examined, a third, "gray", understanding, which makes the epistemological blurriness that already exists more thought-provoking, stands out. The study points out that this hybrid approach, which makes the subject relatively more complicated, differs completely from the "black" view in terms of from whom or where to expect the return of altruistic behavior, but reveals clearer boundaries than the "white" view. As a matter of fact, although this understanding accepts that altruistic behavior is realized with an expectation, it is seen that the addressee of this expectation is based on the understanding that it is not the person or the community that receives the sacrifice but a completely different motivator and a different source of power. In other words, according to the "gray" view, it is accepted that there is an expectation that motivates the individual to act altruistically as in the "black" view, and it is essential not to expect a return from the person who is the subject of the sacrifice as emphasized by the "white" view. That is, the person acts voluntarily [22].

Some critical points can be mentioned when talking about altruism. Some studies have shown that personality is not effective in attitudes towards organ donation, but altruistic nature affects attitudes towards it [23].

People who volunteer to be a living donor with a completely altruistic attitude, without expecting anything in return, make a great sacrifice. Whether the approach of donors is really altruistic in organ transplantation requires a good ethical evaluation.

3.2 Components of altruism

Cognitive framework and processing, religious beliefs and expectations, worldview, empathy, and self-perception determine the altruistic approach. The meaning conveyed by a statement can be defined as the cognitive meaning as the type of meaning that stands directly opposite to the emotional meaning that reveals people's feelings and emotional responses. In the cognitive framework and processing, the process involving the knowing activity with intellectual knowledge refers to activities, such as thinking, grasping, and reasoning and mental behaviors, such as symbolization, belief, and problem-solving [24].

Religious assessment is an assessment of depth, sophistication, and holiness. Religion is a matter of hearing certain things, believing in them, and engaging in certain voluntary activities according to them.

When studies conducted with living donors are examined, it is stated that religious beliefs cause a strong motivation in the donation of kidneys in relatives and non-relative donors. The donation decision of the donor must be examined in detail. Minimal risk to the donor and maximal benefit to the recipient should be the primary objective. The weight of religious elements in the altruistic approach should also be determined.

World view: It is the body of beliefs, thoughts, and attitudes of an individual or a group of people about humanity, future, or similar matters. The most powerful element for donors has been identified as "helping others". Whether the recipient is a relative or not, the donor believes that there will be an increase in self-respect by donating organs.

However, those who accept the help, that is, organ recipients, may feel guilty and indebted. They do not want their donors to be harmed. Feeling guilty about what we do or do not do, say or do not say is another way of wasting time unnecessarily [1].

Patients in need of kidney transplantation experience a long and troublesome process. It seems that most of the donors have witnessed this process. For most donors, not being a donor in this shared life would be 'heartbreaking' for the recipient.

Besides, the fact that the dialysis process reaches an intolerable position and the reflection of this in words motivates the donor to apply to a transplant center as quickly as possible.

Taking the altruistic approach as a basis in organ donation; for example, the kidney may have been reserved for

1. a loved one or a relative within the scope of direct donation,
2. anyone on the general waiting list, or
3. a recipient that has already been qualified.

The donors' actions can be based on individual autonomy and an altruistic approach. Undoubtedly, regarding the decision expressed, in addition to the freedom and decision-making competence expressed by Beauchamp and Childress, the interviews about the choice in terms of the donor, as emphasized by Appelbaum and Grisso, the information provided, awareness of the current situation, and the information given should be reviewed and the deficiencies - if any - must be completed [1].

4. Volunteering

The word 'voluntary' comes from the Old French word 'voluntaire', which was derived from 'voluntarius', whose Latin root is 'voluntas'. The root of the word 'voluntary' is 'voluntas', meaning 'will' in Latin, which means that the individual undertakes a task with their own will and wish. On the other hand, as the Oxford English Dictionary states, what is 'voluntary' is a phenomenon that is 'not restricted or reminded or suggested by someone else's assistance'. 'Volunteer' is also used for 'deliberate action' and when it is used for gifts, it means giving freely or spontaneously to another person [25].

Volunteer in the current Turkish Dictionary of the Turkish Language Association is defined as "a person who willingly undertakes to do a job without any obligation". In the context of consent, "volunteering" refers to the right of a person to make personal decisions independent of the influence of any internal and external factors. In the Dictionary of Bioethics Terms, volunteering is defined as the situation of a person who decides to do a job with their free will and does it without waiting for anything in return. In volunteering, there should not be any force, obligation, or pressure that drives a person. Respect for individual autonomy is the basis of volunteering. Volunteering is considered an ethical basis in medicine, especially in organ transplantation [8]. Ethically, volunteering is one of the basic elements of informed consent. The "volunteer person" must have the characteristics of the person authorized to give informed consent (sound mind) defined by law. Volunteering should be analyzed in the presence of appropriate and adequate information and the absence of psychological coercion and external pressure. From this point of view, we see that the conditions related to volunteering are in parallel with the conditions required for autonomous action [1]. Not only do medical or psychosocial factors play a role in the selection process by living donors, but every medical professional, lawyer or ethicist agrees that the decision to donate must be voluntary and informed. However, proving the determination of volunteering is not always easy; it requires intense effort. For the consent to be meaningful, the process must also be carried out in a meaningful way. In other words, consent must be voluntary. This is not a surprising statement and everyone agrees that volunteering is important. However, it should not be forgotten that volunteering is a concept that can be quickly overlooked and create a dangerous situation in the daily practice of medicine.

Although organ donations from living donors are commendable, it should not be forgotten that they are considered voluntary. For living donors to make sure they do not make inappropriate decisions within their own values and views on self-sacrifice, risk, or similar topics, transplant teams need to present the criteria they use to select living donors to the community. For policies and practices supporting living donations to be morally acceptable, they should not turn into a means of influence or pressure [7]. In this sense, the concept of volunteering or the opposite, reluctance, is important.

In the evaluation of whether a person is a volunteer for organ donation, there are signs that appear not only in words but also in behaviors and give us clues in determining volunteering; for example, the donor comes for the tests alone, tries to learn the results, does not lean his head forward when the organ donation decision is made, or insists on being a donor, etc. [26]. But what exactly is volunteering?

Stating that the action of a voluntary person is the product of the will of the person acting in the light of the concepts of knowledge, freedom, and volunteering, Babor divides volunteering into thirteen types or degrees. In terms of organ transplantation, it is necessary to examine perfect/imperfect, direct/indirect, and positive/negative volunteering concepts. Perfect volunteering is defined as an action taken with full knowledge and consent. Imperfect volunteering is the opposite of this concept, and there are flaws in both knowledge and consent. Direct volunteering expresses a voluntary action that is desired as an end in itself. In indirect volunteering, on the other hand, the action is not an end in itself but is desired as an anticipated result or sequence of action. Positive volunteering mentions the volunteering present in performing an action, while in negative volunteering, the person avoids the action [27]. For the person's action to be considered voluntary in organ donation, it should be an action that includes all characteristics of perfect, direct, and positive volunteering.

In an ethical guide prepared for the assessment of living organ donors, the evaluation of whether the person is a volunteer or not is checked from 10 different angles. The guide addresses issues, such as potential donor's psycho-social status, financial status, relationship with the transplant candidate, the reason for donation, the conditions under which the decision has been made and by whom the potential donor is asked to donate, the convenience of the potential donor to refuse the donation request, the comfort of the potential donor near other family members, proof of material reward for the donation, willingness and motivation of the potential donor, and the imbalance of power between the potential living donor and the recipient [28].

The concept of volunteering may be affected by some positive and negative factors. In this sense, it is useful to look at these factors.

4.1 Positive and negative factors affecting volunteering

The "gift" that the recipient receives from the donor free of charge, which has no physical or symbolic equivalent by nature, is so extraordinary that as a result, the donor, recipient, and their families may find themselves in a mutual creditor-debtor spiral. Such a situation also describes the importance of volunteering in organ donation. It is essential for the organ donor to donate in full volunteering and to be completely free from negative factors. Also, informed consent for organ transplantation requires sufficient information sharing for both the patient and the organ and tissue donor and communication that is free from coercion and threat, does not involve persuasion, and does not aim to manipulate the decision.

It is clear that there is a non-altruistic motivation if the person requests a reward for a donation. However, the fact that such a demand has accompanying elements does not mean that the donation is motivated by altruism and that it involves an altruistic approach. One of the three pillars of autonomy is that the individual is far from influences that control them. In other words, for the action to be autonomous, the person should not be in a situation that prevents their self-management either by internal or external forces. However, not all effects on the person by others are controlling. In this section, controlling concepts will be discussed.

Evaluating the determinants of attitudes towards organ removal from the dead, willingness to donate, and donor behavior in a systematic review of 33 published studies, Wakefield et al. emphasizes that individuals' attitudes towards donation are complex due to differences in social norms, existing laws, and interactions between beliefs and individual factors in each country [29].

However, apart from these regional and personal differences, there are factors that affect donation positively and negatively. A study shows that the team, which will talk to the family of the deceased during the donation process, should reassure the family with their linguistic and cognitive abilities and show their emotions, which has a significant effect on whether the family is a donor [30].

Although organ donation is apparently supported by society, the level of organ donation is very low. Psychological factors that affect the person's decisions to become a donor also play a role in this complexity. They have also led to the need to understand how people predict or inhibit the desire to become organ donors. In a study conducted by Morgan et al., it has been shown that the perceived benefits of organ donation play an effective role in the decision-making process [31]. The volunteer choices of potential donors (e.g., women in strong patriarchal cultures) who do not understand that they are an autonomous moral person, act as expected, and never dare to reject are undermined by persuasion, encouragement, and pressure.

In determining whether an action is autonomous, the two most important conditions require that the person fully understands the issue and is not under control. There is a gradual transition from total freedom to total control for the status of both understanding and being free of controlling influences. This transition involves the scales that reveal the "autonomous actions" and "non-autonomous actions" domains. By considering these domains and thresholds for specific purposes, the boundary between "autonomous enough" and "not autonomous enough" can be carefully determined [7]. There are some factors, such as requests, family, or legal obligations, in making personal decisions. But there are also some factors other than these factors that will directly affect the person's ability to act autonomously. All of these factors are detrimental to the autonomy of the person and aim at taking the person under control.

Informed consent is the most important issue in ensuring the autonomy of the person. Instead of reading standard forms, each individual's unique needs for information should be taken into account with a "customized" approach. It would not be wrong to state that the dignity and value of the human being, the principle of autonomy, and legal aspects of organ transplantation should be addressed for each person in the informed consent form [32].

Concepts such as sacrifice, compassion, interest, renunciation, loyalty, reliability, concern, respect and justice, empathy, and emotional ties are among the positive factors that affect volunteering. Besides, the altruistic nature of the person is an important issue that requires research on its own among positive factors.

Volunteering is essential for autonomous action. External control over an individual's actions weakens the voluntary nature of the actions. Such effects can be grouped under three main categories, namely, persuasion, coercion, and manipulation. If we detail these concepts, we can better evaluate the negative factors affecting volunteering.

4.1.1 Persuasion

Persuasion is the effort or process of encouraging people to change their current beliefs, values, or attitudes, or to gain new ones. This extremely complex process may be based on rational discussions or messages or it may include a method that addresses irrational desires or needs [33]. The process of persuasion is typically analyzed in terms of who said what, how, and with what effect, and expresses whether any attitude changes have occurred [34]. Valapour explains persuasion as influencing by using reasoning and states that when the person is persuaded, they freely accept the effect; therefore, they think it is an ethically acceptable action and that it does not undermine the voluntary nature of the person and they regard it as compatible with autonomous actions [35]. Hançerlioğlu handles the concept of persuasion under the heading of "deceiving" and defines it as "making something accepted with mental evidence or making someone believe" [36]. However, it is seen that the meaning of the concept of "volunteering" has not been fully understood. There are also studies showing that people's attitudes towards organ donation can be changed with persuasion and manipulation techniques [37].

Persuasion arises as a result of the reasoning offered to a person to believe something is worth believing. Inviting people to be reasonable and addressing people's feelings are different situations [7]. In summary, persuasion is the process of making a person believe something that they did not believe at the outset.

4.1.2 Pressure /threat/force/coercion

Hançerlioğlu states that pressure leads to a situation that prevents free development naturally and socially and that it prevents free behavior [36]. Budak defines pressure as forcing the person to act one way or another and as excessive or stress-causing expectations from the person and states that what is felt as pressure changes depending on the person or education level [33].

Coercion exists when a person poses a credible and serious threat of harm or coercion in an attempt to control another person. Whether the pressure will occur or not depends on how the target person will receive this threat, and this response varies from person to person. Coercion occurs when the perpetrator behind a person's actions is not their own free will and their conscious behavior about areas in which they are knowledgeable ceases to be autonomous when they receive a credible threat [7]. It is the pressure that causes a person to act contrary to their will under a threat of harm. The threat of harm is an essential component of the concept of coercion, and a forced action reflects someone else's choices, not one's own choices, as it is based on a credible threat. Therefore, decisions made under coercion and actions carried out are not autonomous.

Following the coercion, the person makes their own decision. Therefore, although it is said that this, in a sense, is an autonomous choice and should be stated as a voluntary act, this kind of volunteering is volunteering that is not perfect, indirect, and negative. Therefore, as mentioned at the beginning, it is not a desired situation for organ donation. In terms of organ donation, the decision to be made after coercion, pressure or threat is not an autonomous and consensual choice.

Coercion entails a real, convincing, and intended threat that pushes a person into unwanted action and pushes his autonomy out of self-control. In this sense, threat involves applying force to a person to do something or to restrict their freedom. In principle, threat requires a genuine, reliable, intended, and willing orientation [26]. In these concepts, which we generally express, there is a use of physical or psychological force against the autonomy of the person. The plan of bringing the person to the level to do the desired thing lies at the heart of applying pressure, threat, force, and coercion.

Studies on the psychosocial effect of living kidney donation indicate that many living donors believe that the decision to donate is not a real choice and that they feel compelled to donate [38, 39]. In a similar study conducted in the USA, 40% of the donors who donated living organs between 2002 and 2005 reported that they felt some pressure to donate [40]. Understanding volunteer donation only as the absence of coercion will indicate a narrow meaning as it does not cover more sophisticated interventions such as persuasion and manipulation. In this sense, it is necessary to examine the concept of manipulation among the negative factors that affect volunteering.

4.1.3 Manipulation

The concept of manipulation increasingly plays a central role in debates about free will and moral responsibility. Manipulation is essentially the orientation of the person to do what the manipulator wants by means other than persuasion or coercion. In this sense, manipulation encompasses some forms of influence that are neither persuasion nor coercion/threat/force. The most likely type of manipulation in healthcare is informational. It is the presentation of information in such a way that the person is directed to do what the manipulator wants by understanding the situation differently. In this sense, informational manipulation is also against autonomy. Hiding certain information, telling lies, or exaggerating the meaning or importance of certain information to make people believe in unfounded things are the kinds of actions that can harm autonomous choices.

Manipulation is the deliberate and successful influence on the available choices one can make, either by non-coercively altering or by changing one's perception of those choices. "Being manipulated" is subjective in nature and depends on the person's reaction [35]. If the living donor accepts surgical intervention because of its benefits, they must also accept the possible risks. This is not a manipulative situation [26].

It is a fact that some living organ donors are also manipulated with financial support. Besides, due to the paternalistic approach of the physician to their recipient patient, they may attempt to manipulate the living donor candidate to affect their willingness. The assessment of the living donor candidate by a different transplant team is necessary so that the manipulation that may occur can be evaluated.

5. Conclusion

Organ transplantation is not an issue limited to health. It is also a field of both law and ethics as a medical practice surrounded by social, cultural and value problems which have challenging solution. The applicability of every medical practice in the clinic is within the limits determined by the law, and there are laws that vary by countries regarding organ transplantation. The fact that concepts such as human rights, right to health, human value, bodily integrity, and quality of life are predominantly handled within philosophy is also a guide in the preparation of existing legal texts. One of the main points that everyone agrees on is the value of life and that it is an inalienable personality right. The right to life is defined as the existence of a healthy and complete body and the ability to continue lives by protecting them against potential threats and dangers. The right to life is also directly linked to human dignity. While the material aspect of the right to life is expressed with the content of protecting the bodily integrity of the person and not being exposed to bad behavior, living under humane living conditions also emphasizes the spiritual aspect of the right in question. Debates about organ transplantation arise between the right to life and the right to determine one's own future. For example, obtaining a kidney from a potential donor is very important in saving the life of the terminal kidney patient who will die. Without harming the bodily functions, the living donor will use their ethical right to give up their organ that is valuable for them but can also be lived without. In this context, medical evaluations of the donor and the recipient alone will not be enough. It is also necessary to examine how altruistic behavior leads to volunteerism. For people to live a good life they have determined for themselves, they must not interfere with the autonomy of others. Especially, it is necessary to evaluate carefully whether the living donors in the family donate with a mission to save or because they are really volunteers. Saving lives can be a commendable option when one can be sure of the willingness of living donors. If we accept that voluntary donation is a moral and legal requirement, the issues of persuasion, coercion, force, lack of financial incentives, and manipulation and non-instrumentalization of individuals need to be addressed in a more systematic and detailed manner. The scales to be used to determine the volunteering in organ transplantation will contribute to the informed consent processes of health professionals, as well as basing the right to determine one's own future and right to life on the self-worth of the individual.

Author details

Mesut Güvenbaş and Omur Sayligil*
Department of History of Medicine and Ethics, Faculty of Medicine, Eskişehir Osmangazi University, Eskişehir, Turkey

*Address all correspondence to: sayligil@ogu.edu.tr

IntechOpen

© 2021 The Author(s). Licensee IntechOpen. This chapter is distributed under the terms of the Creative Commons Attribution License (http://creativecommons.org/licenses/by/3.0), which permits unrestricted use, distribution, and reproduction in any medium, provided the original work is properly cited.

References

[1] Elçioğlu Ö. Böbrek Naklinde Canlı Vericiler: Gönüllülüğü Belirlemede Puanlama ve Derecelendirme Modeli Önerisi, In: Erdemir, A.D. et al. editors. Organ ve Doku Naklinde Tıp Etiği ve Tıp Hukuku Sorunları, I. Uluslararası Tıp Etiği ve Tıp Hukuku Kongresi Bildiri Kitabı. İstanbul: Nobel Tıp Kitabevleri; 2007. p. 33-53.

[2] Biller-Andorno N. Voluntariness in Living-Related Organ Donation. Transplantation. 2011;92(6):617-619. DOI: 10.1097/TP.0b013e3182279120

[3] Al-Khader A.A. A Model for Scoring And Grading Willingness of a Potential Living Related Donor. J.Med.Ethics; 2005;31: 338-340. DOI: 10.1136/jme.2004.009282

[4] Wright L, Faith K, Richardson R, Grant D. Ethical Guidelines for the Evaluation of Living Organ Donors. J. Can. Chir. 2004;47(6):408-413.

[5] The Authors for the Live Organ Donor Consensus Group. Consensus Statement on the Live Organ Donor. JAMA, 2000;284(22):2919-2926. DOI: 10.1001/jama.284.22.2919.

[6] Irodat. [Internet] Available from: https://www.irodat.org/?p=database [Accessed: 2020-08-29]

[7] Beauchamp T.L, Childress, J.F. *Biyomedikal Etik Prensipleri*. Translated by: M. Kemal Temel. İstanbul: BETİM; 2017. 82, 158-159, 210-211, 307-315 pp.

[8] Oğuz, Y.N, Tepe H, Örnek Büken N, Kırımsoy Kucur D. Biyoetik Terimleri Sözlüğü. 1st ed. Ankara: Türkiye Felsefe Kurumu; 2005. 115, 197-199, 256 pp.

[9] Monreo K.R. The Heart of Altruism. Perception of a Common Humanity. Princeton: Princeton University Pres.1996; 6-23 pp.

[10] Dictionary [Internet]. Available from: http://www.merriam-webster.com/dictionary/ altruism [Accessed: 2020-08-16]

[11] Dictionary [Internet]. Available from: www.tdk.gov.tr [Accessed: 2020-07-10]

[12] Wright L, Ross K, Abbey S, Levy G, Grant D. Living Anonimous Liver Donation Case Report and Ethical Justification. Am J.of Transplantation. 2007;7:1032-1035. DOI: 10.1111/j.1600-6143.2006.01725.x

[13] Kropotkin P.A. Karşılıklı Yardımlaşma. Evrimin Bir Faktörü. İstanbul: Kaos Yayınevi; 2001.

[14] Bierhoff H.W. Prosocial Behaviour. [Internet]. Available from: https://www.blackwellpublishing.com/content/hewstonesocialpsychology/chapters/cpt9.pdf [Accessed: 2020-11-11]

[15] Batson C. D. Altruism in Humans. New York: Oxford University Press; 2011. 1-19 pp.

[16] Tomini F. Transferring to family and friends: A review of the Motives, Evidence, and the role of Economics. [Working Papers]. Netherlands: Maastricht Graduate School of Governance; 2010.

[17] Hazlitt H. Ahlakın Temelleri. The Foundation of Morality. Translated by: Aydın M, Tapramaz R. Ankara: Liberte Yayınları; 2006. 114-116 pp.

[18] Vugt M. V, Roberts G, Hardy C. Competitive Altruism: A Theory of Reputation-Based Cooperation in Groups. In: Dunbar R.I.M, Barrett L. editors. The Oxford Handbook of Evolutionary Psychology. New York: Oxford University Press; 2007. 531-543 pp.

[19] Ashton M. C, Paunonen S. V, Hekmes E, Jackson D. N. Kin Altruism, Reciprocal Altruism, and Big Five Personality Factors. Evolution and Human Behaviour. 1998; 19:243-255. DOI: 10.1016/S1090-5138(98)00009-9

[20] Nijkamp M. D, Hollestelle M. L, Zeegers M. P, Van den Borne B, Reubsaet A. To be (come) or not to be (come) an organ donor, that's the question: A meta-analysis of determinant and intervention studies. Health Psychology Review. 2008;2(1):20-40. DOI: 10.1080/17437190802307971

[21] Batson C. D. Prosocial Motivation: Is it Ever Truly altruistic? In: Berkowitz L. editör. Advances in experimentalsocial psychology, Volume: 20. San Diego, CA: Academic Press; 1987:65-122.

[22] Yeşilkaya M. Özgeci Davranış Olgusuna İlişkin Epistemolojik Sorunlar Üzerine Bir İnceleme: Siyah, Beyaz ve Gri. Manas Sosyal Araştırmalar Dergisi. 2018;7(4):469-489.

[23] Hill E.M. Posthumous Organ Donation Attitudes, Intentions to Donate, and Organ Donor Status: Examining the Role of the Big Five Personality Dimensions and Altruism. Personality and Individual Differences. 2016;88:182-186. DOI: 10.1016/j.paid.2015.09.021

[24] Cevizci A. Felsefe Sözlüğü. İstanbul: Paradigma Yayınları. 2002. 800 p.

[25] Hogg M. Voluntariness and Consent. In: Obligations: Law and Language, Cambridge: Cambridge University Press. 2017;269-304. DOI: 10.1017/9781316104415.008

[26] Elçioğlu Ö, Duman S. Concept of the Voluntariness in Kidney Transplantation from the Position of Donors and Recipients. In: Chiarelli B. editör. Global Bioethics-Perspective for Human Survival. Intechopen; 2011. p. 99-128. DOI: 10.5772/18487

[27] Babor E.R. Ethics The Philosophical Discipline of Action, Updated Ed. Manila: Rex Book Store; 2007. 164-167 pp.

[28] University Health Network Bioethics Program. Ethical Guidelines fort he Evaluation of Living Organ Donors. Toronto: University Health Network. 2016. 8 p.

[29] Wakefield C.E, Watts K.J, Homewood J, Meiser B, Siminoff L.A. Attitudes Toward Organ Donation and Donor Behavior: A Review of the Internation Literature. Progress in Transplantation. 2010;20(4):380-391. DOI: 10.7182/prtr.20.4.p54651601pg80183

[30] Schwartz K. Decoding the Ideal Organ Donation Requestor. [thesis]. USA: University of the Rockies; 2012.

[31] Morgan S.E, Stephenson M.T, Harrison T.R, Afifi W.A, Long S.D. Feelings: How Rational is the Decision to Become an Organ Donor?, Journal of Health Psychology. 2008;13:644-658. DOI: 10.1177/1359105308090936

[32] Güvenbaş M, Şaylıgil Ö. Bilgilendirilmiş Rıza İçin Akılcı Bir Dizi Standarda Gerek Var mıdır?. Türkiye Klinikleri J.Med.Ethics. 2019;27(3):277-284. DOI: 10.5336/mdethic.2018-62938

[33] Budak S. Psikoloji Sözlüğü. Ankara: Bilim ve Sanat Yayınları; 2000. 110, 392 p.

[34] Petty R.E. The Role of Cognitive Responses in Attitude Change Processes. In: Petty R.E, Ostrom T.M, Brock T.C, editors. Cognitive responses in persuasion. Hillsdale, NJ: Lawrence Erlbaum Associates; 1981. p. 135-139.

[35] Valapour M. The Live Organ Donor's Consent: Is It Informed and Voluntary?

Transplantation Reviews. 2008;22:196-199. DOI: 10.1016/j.trre.2008.02.004

[36] Hançerlioğlu O. Felsefe Ansiklopedisi Kavramlar ve Akımlar, 4. ed. İstanbul: Remzi Kitabevi; 2005. Vol 1:136; Vol 3: 202.

[37] Julka D.L, Marsh K.L. An Attitude Functions Approach to Increasing Organ-Donation Participation. Journal of Applied Social Psychology. 2005;35(4):821-849. DOI: 10.1111/j.1559-1816.2005.tb02148.x

[38] Eggeling C. The Psychosocial Implications of Live-Related Kidney Donation. The European Dialysis and Transplant Nurses Association/ European Renal Care Association. 1999;25:19-22.

[39] Lennerling A, Forsberg A, Nyberg G. Becoming a Living Kidney Donor. Transplantation. 2003;76:1243-1247.

[40] Valapour M, Kahn J.P, Bailey R, Matas A.J. Assessing Elements of Informed Consent Among Living Donors. Clin. Transplant. 2011;25(2):185-190. DOI: 10.1111/j.1399-0012.2010.01374.x

Chapter 8

Future Prospects of Organ Transplantation

Mehmet Nur Altinörs

Abstract

The gap between organ demand and supply is an universal problem in organ and tissue transplantation therapy. The gap is growing in spite of efforts spent in medical, educational, social areas and mass media support. This reality has created the need for completely new therapeutic alternatives for the management of end-stage organ disease. The present research should continue in future aiming to discover systems and devices capable of totally replacing the traditional transplantation. On the other hand, a different progress in underway in transplantation. The indication for solid organ transplantation is to save life and promote quality of life. The new developing transplantations of composite tissue, uterus and face are performed with completely different indications. Facial defects caused by various insults cause serious functional and esthetic disorders, psychological and social problems. Facial transplant surgery is accomplished to overcome such problems. Uterus transplantation is emerging as an alternative to female infertility. Transplantation of composite tissue includes different organs. The main purpose of composite tissue transplantation is to restore reduced or completely lost functions and to increase the quality of life. Nerve regeneration must occur as a consequence of transplant to regain sensory and motor functions. It appears that the future of transplantation involves developments in two main streams; invention of completely new tools for solid organ transplantation and advances in the transplantation of different organs including uterus, face and composite tissue.

Keywords: composite tissue, facial, solid organ, transplantation, uterus

1. Introduction

The idea of replacing a malfunctioning diseased organ by the same organ dates back to antiquity, but major inventions and successful practice of transplanting solid organs have occurred in the second half of the 20th century. Pioneering work in human-to-human organ transplantation started in the 1950's and in following decade. Since then, improvements in surgical techniques, better postoperative management in the intensive care units, the introduction of brain death concept and its beneficial effect of enlarging the donor pool, a better understanding of the natural course of the various diseases leading to organ failure, new immunosuppressive agents have all contributed to transplantation activities. Today organ transplantation is a definitive treatment for an end-stage disease with low morbidity and mortality rates. Efforts directed to the education of medical staff and the general public, controlled system of financial payment for the living donor, similarly gifting to deceased donor's family, extending the donor criteria,

IntechOpen

acceptance of paired organ donation, organ donation campaigns and media support are among the other measures to promote transplantation.

2. Discussion

Organ transplantation is a definitive and curative treatment for end-stage organ disease. The preferred source of organs is from the deceased. Particularly in developing countries, organ harvesting is more from living donors. Although the morbidity and mortality rates for living donors are extremely low, completely healthy individuals are exposed to medical, surgical, psychological and sometimes to economic risks.

While organ transplantation will continue to be the definitive treatment for the present and foreseen future, the statistical evidence revealing the gap between demand and supply and the experience of the global medical community has clearly shown that even the centers with best figures of organ supply are far from meeting the growing need. Therefore the scientific world has arrived at a point to think and search for alternative solutions and different therapeutic modalities for end-stage organ diseases. An overview of the present state of organ transplantation suggests that future interest and work will be focused on three major points:

a. increasing the frequency, safety and outcome of traditional transplantation activities. This would cover research to discover ways of expanding donor pool, especially cadaveric, and innovative work for longer and safer preservation of harvested organs and methods that would help to obtain better graft and survival rates. Weissenbacher and associates have reported the beneficial effects of ex-vivo/ex-situ hypothermic and normothermic machine perfusion in the transplantation of liver, kidney, intestine and pancreas. The beneficial effects include viability, organ utilization and improved initial graft function. The authors have considered the potential role of normothermic regional perfusion to re-condition donors after circulatory death organs before retrieval. Machine perfusion presents superiority over the traditional cold preservation method. Since organ preservation is an essential aspect of the transplantation process, these developments provide hope for better organ quality and longer viability [1].

In solid-organ transplant, cell therapy is used as an immunomodulation therapy or as a functioning graft. The beneficial effects of cell therapy in solid-organ transplantation are long-term kidney allograft survival and avoiding the well-known adverse effects of immunosuppressive drugs. Cell-based therapy in solid organ transplant is indicated for the treatment of ischemic reperfusion injury, for the prevention of chronic allograft nephropathy and induction of long-term allograft tolerance. Immunoregulatory cells act when it is necessary for immune suppression and there are several mechanisms by many pharmacologic targets [2].

b. developments in relatively new, emerging transplantations including the uterus, face and composite tissue. Such transplantations are expected to be performed with increasing frequency.

c. the ultimate goal of producing completely new devices or bioartificial organs which eventually would replace organ transplantation and maintain immunosuppressive free life. Nowadays may be considered as the transition period where devices can at least partially take over the functions of the failing organ and bridge patients to transplantation.

3. Xenotransplantation

Xenotransplantation, not a new concept in this field, is a controversial issue. Xenotransplantation which means transplantation of an organ, tissue, or cells between two different species, has regained attention because of advantages such as rich source, the chance of planned, and multiple transplantations. The main disadvantages are the possibility of animal disease transmission, immunologic, and physiologic differences.

In the sixteenth- century animal blood has been transferred to humans. Skin, corneal and blood vessel xenotransplantations were the early attempts. The kidney was the first solid organ of xenotransplantation. Dr. Keith Reemtsma, working at Tulane University, performed 13 xenotransplants in the 1960's using both chimpanzee kidneys on each surgery. Only one patient survived for nine months while the rest died within 4 to 8 weeks due to either infection or rejection. Dr. Thomas Starzl performed the first liver xenotransplant using baboons as donors [3].

In October 1984, orthotopic cardiac xenotransplantation on " Baby Fae" was performed by Dr. Leonard Bailey and his co-workers. The recipient was a 12-day neonate harboring hypoplastic left heart syndrome. The donor was an immunologically-selected baboon. The baby died on the 20th postoperative day. Neither humoral nor cellular rejection of the xenograft was noted [4].

Galactosyl-α-1-3, galactose [GAL] is the most important antigen in xenotransplantation. GAL is expressed in most cells of all mammals except humans, including porcine. GAL is found in intestinal bacteria, and there are antibodies against GAL in humans. Antibodies to nonGAL antigens are still a problem. The primary methods to prevent hyperacute rejection are the elimination of antibodies by plasmapheresis and immunoadsorption and depletion or inhibition of complements [5].

In the last 30 years, researchers have determined that the pig is the most suitable animal for xenotransplantation. The reasons for this are short maturation time, the human similarity in size and physiological aspects, and low risk of animal disease transmission. Genetically modified pigs have been developed to overcome the molecular incompatibility between species. Another important step is the development of "knockout" pigs lacking the 1,3 galactosyl transferase gene encoding enzymes responsible for immunologic expression. Genetic engineering techniques can be easily applied to create rejection-resistant pig organs [6].

Knockout pigs have contributed to prolonged survival particularly in heart and kidney transplantation. Survival of pig-to-nonhuman primate heterotopic heart, kidney, and islet xenotransplantation over 900 days, over 400 days, and over 600 days respectively has been reported [7]. Bioartificial organs that contain pig cells or tissues have gained considerable clinical experience and the risks have been reduced [8]. For the time being, the indications of xenografting seem unclear but should be kept aside for exceptional cases.

4. Rare organ transplants

4.1 Composite tissue transplantation

When body structures composed of multiple tissues derived from ectoderm and endoderm is transplanted then the procedure is named composite tissue allotransplantation. Such transplants are also known as " vascular composite allografts". The concept of composite tissue transplantation includes hand, face, larynx, joint, abdominal wall transplantations. This type of transplant has a life-changing nature, as the main goal is to restore reduced or completely lost functions and to increase the quality of life. Unlike solid organ transplants, nerve regeneration must occur in the transplant to restore sensory and motor functions.

The first hand transplant was tried in Ecuador in 1964 with failure. The failure was believed to be associated with inadequate immunosuppression [9]. Dubernard and his coworkers transplanted the right distal forearm and hand from a deceased donor to a 48- year- old male patient who had had a traumatic amputation of the distal third of his right forearm. Motor and sensory recovery were evaluated as excellent six months postoperatively and no serious signs of rejection were observed [10].

The same group performed surgical intervention involving bone fixation, arterial and venous anastomosis, nerve suturing, tendon, and muscle joining in a 33-year old, bilateral forearm amputated patient. They applied physical therapy, electrostimulation, and occupational therapy in the postoperative period. In the postoperative 15th month, they observed satisfactory sensory and motor improvement as well as improvement in the quality of life. This procedure was the first human double-hand transplantation with satisfactory results [11]. It is generally believed that bilateral below-elbow amputation is the most accepted indication for hand transplantation.

In a study comparing the functional and psychosocial outcomes of hand transplantation and prosthesis options, upper extremity functions were globally evaluated with ARAT [Action Research Arm Test] and SHAP [Southampton Hand Assessment Procedure]. The study revealed that functional results are not significantly different. The advantages of transplantation are that it provides sensory and self-perception in addition to providing motor activity. Complications due to immunosuppression pose a disadvantage in transplantation. However, if immunosuppression is well tolerated, regeneration of an organ with its like is naturally an advantage. In bilateral below-elbow amputees, it is understood that the benefit is greater when the acquisition of motor and sensory functions is compared with the risks of immunosuppression. Unilateral amputees can compensate for many functional deficits by using healthy limbs and prostheses. Also, In addition, there is no need for a long-term rehabilitation program after prosthesis implantation, as in transplantation. For these reasons, the prosthesis option is a priority in patients with unilateral below-elbow amputees [12].

4.2 Facial transplant

Facial defects caused by congenital malformations, gunshot injuries, animal bites, burns, traumas, or tumors such as neurofibromatosis cause serious functional and esthetic disorders, psychological and social problems. Basic requirements for a successful face transplant are craniofacial and microsurgical techniques, triple immunosuppression therapy, intensive physical therapy, and psychological support initiated in the early postoperative period for functions such as smelling, eating, drinking, laughing and speaking. In surgery, maxillary and facial branches of the external carotid artery are used for arterial anastomoses. Facial, external jugular and thyrolingofacial veins are preferred for venous anastomoses. Vascular anastomoses are followed by nerve anastomoses. The most problematic aspects of surgery are prolonged anesthesia, excessive blood loss, and transfusions to replace this loss, complex vascular anatomy due to trauma and changes related to previous reconstructive surgeries [13].

Since the surgical experience with facial transplantation is limited, there are no algorithms on long-term results, late complications and their management. In a study conducted to clarify these issues and to get the opinions of physicians experienced in face transplantation, the training of the recipient, how to define the failure in facial transplant, approach to complications and their management were investigated. Approximately 30% of those who received a survey responded. While 93.8% of the participants stated that facial transplant failure, 91.1% mortality, and 78.8% chronic organ rejection are the points that should be discussed, the answers revealed that there is no consensus about the definition of mortality rates and facial transplantation. Also, it has been observed that even in centers with experience in facial transplantation, there are no protocols for the treatment of rejection in the chronic period [14].

The first partial facial transplant was performed in Amiens France with success. The patient was a victim of dog bite thus losing lips, nose and, central cheeks. The patient had recovered sensory and motor for a long period of time [15]. Immunosuppressive therapy complications and graft rejection, which are common problems in all organ transplants, are valid in face transplantation, and also a case diagnosed with beta-cell lymphoma and eventually developing chronic graft rejection has been reported [16]. Squamous cell carcinoma developed in the fourth case of face transplant performed by Dr. Özkan and his associates. After treatment, severe infection, respiratory failure and allograft rejection developed. Despite the removal of the graft, the patient was lost [17].

Future progress in face transplantation can be achieved with the contribution of different fields of science and technology. Naturally this holds true for the progress of other organ transplantations. These include tissue engineering, creation of functional autogenous-mucosal-cutaneous junctions, neural regeneration, 3-D printed bioresorbable scaffolds, and elimination of antigenic transplanted tissue [18]. The drawbacks of facial transplantation are the cost, relatively small number of potential recipients and only cadaveric donation.

4.3 Uterus transplant

Uterus transplantation has emerged as an alternative solution for female infertility. The first success in uterine transplantation was to ensure pregnancy by replantation of the uterus and ovaries in dogs [19].

The first example of human application was a live uterine transplant in Saudi Arabia on April 2000, to a 26-year old woman who lost her uterus six years ago due to postpartum hemorrhage. The donor was 46-year old lady. The patient had acute vascular thrombosis 99 days after transplant and had a hysterectomy. Although acute thrombosis and infarction were detected in the vessels in macroscopic and microscopic examination of the excised uterus, no findings suggesting rejection were found [20]. An important milestone in uterine transplantation is the allograft uterine transplant performed to a 23-year-old woman diagnosed with Mayer-Rokitansky-Kuster-Hauser syndrome in 2011 at Akdeniz University, Turkey. Embryo transfer was provided 18 months after transplantation and live birth was not possible although clinical pregnancy was detected by transvaginal ultrasound [21].

The first clinical applications in Sweeden were made with nine living donors. In 2013, uterus transplantation was performed on a 23-year-old woman with congenital absence of uterus [Rokitansky syndrome] at Sahlgrenska University Hospital in Gothenburg, Sweeden. The donor was a living 61-year old lady. The patient, who had a menstruation on the 43rd day after the transplant, continued to have regular menstruation. One year after the transplant, a single embryo transfer resulted in pregnancy. Therefore, the triple immunosuppression was started. The patient, pregnant for 31 weeks and five days, was admitted to the hospital with complaints of preeclampsia and was taken to cesarean section due to abnormal cardiotocography findings. A healthy male baby, with APGAR scores of 9,9,10 and with a weight compatible [1775 gr] with gestational age, was born. Thus, the first live birth was achieved with the uterine transplantation method in the medical literature [22].

Uterine transplantation does not carry a vital indication. Medical, surgical, legal, ethical, psychological, and social aspects of the process are discussed in medical and related communities. Common requirements for recipient and donor are good general health, no history of infection and cancer in the last five years. The upper age limit for the recipient is 35–40 and 55–65 for the donor. In elderly women, it is believed that the vessels be affected by arteriosclerosis, probably due to the atrophic nature of the uterus. The effect of age on graft success is unknown. Among the peroperative problems is the long duration of surgical intervention, especially in the donor.

A characteristic of uterine transplantation is the removal of the transplanted uterus after one or two births to prevent the patient from immunosuppressive therapy for a longer period. This period is foreseen as an average of five years. Therefore, it is not particularly superior to prefer live donors. Besides, psychological problems that the recipient may feel against the donor are eliminated by the use of cadaver uterus. Ethical foundations of uterine transplantation are gathered under the name of Montreal criteria. Accordingly, six conditions should be fulfilled for the recipient, four conditions for the donor, and four conditions for the healthcare team performing the treatment [23].

5. Future prospects

5.1 Organ bioengineering and regenerative medicine

The field of tissue engineering is evolving rapidly and is opening new horizons for novel treatment opportunities. Tissue engineering and regenerative medicine includes artificial and biological materials.

Whole organ decellularization and recellularization have gained importance in recent years. Decellularization, as the name implies, means the removal of all cellular components from the organ and at the same time, the micro and macro anatomy of the extracellular matrix is preserved. These scaffolds are repopulated with patient- derived cells or stem cells to construct an individual specific organ. Consequently immunosuppression is no more needed. Bioreactors are used for decellularization and recellularization [24].

The technology used for organ bioengineering includes seeding cells on supporting scaffolding materials. The cell-scaffold technology uses adult cells, various progenitor cells, and progenitor cells that may differentiate into specific adult cells. Bioreactors are used for uniform scaffold distribution, nutrient supply, and waste removal. The regeneration process takes place in the bioreactors and consequently, bioengineered tissues and organs can be harvested for analysis and implantation. Bioreactors facilitate, monitor, and control biochemical and biophysical processes [25].

Mostly used scaffolds are decellularized allogeneic extracellular matrix which in turn is recellularized by autologous or stem cells. A wide variety of human tissues and organs have been decellularized for tissue engineering. These include cartilage, bone, skeletal muscle, tendon, adipose tissue, heart, arteries and veins, gingiva, cornea, vocal folds, peripheral nerves, intestine, liver, pancreas, kidney, bladder, male and female reproductive systems, products of child birth and complex composite structures. Decellularization requires efficient removal of immunogenic cellular materials and maintenance of nonimmunogenic extracellular matrix. Human tissues are harvested from cadavers and surgery. An advantageous point is the fact that extracellular matrix derived from decellularization of a certain tissue may be used for tissue engineering of another tissue type [26].

Organ bioengineering aims to develop extracorporeal systems to compensate or completely replace the functions of a diseased organ. As an example, an extracorporeal method designed to substitute liver function should have the capacity to detoxify, synthesize, and regulate. The artificial liver support system has beneficial effects on the prognosis of patients with acute-on-chronic failure. These beneficial effects are generated by improving jaundice, ameliorating hemodynamic instability, reducing portal hypertension, and improving hepatic encephalopathy.

The de-and recellularization technique has been used to produce heart, lung, liver, kidney, and intestine. Despite of some laboratory success, the technique seems to be improved before clinical application [27].

5.2 Bioartificial organs

Dialysis treatment initiated the development of artificial organs. Bioartificial organs are aimed to fully compensate for the functions of a failing organ and they closely mimic human organs. Bioengineering is the mainstay of producing bioartificial organs, but an interdisciplinary approach including the contribution of material science, cell biology, mechanics, chemistry, informatics, surgery, computer science, physics, and medicine is required. Organ manufacturing, in its simplest definition, is producing bioartificial organs using living cells, other material, and advanced processing technologies. Organ manufacturing technologies are basically classified into three groups: fully automated, semi-automated, and hand- manipulated [28].

5.3 3D bioprinting

3D Bioprinting is a rapid prototyping and additive manufacturing technique used to produce artificial implants. Tissue and organ regeneration is one of the fields where 3D bioprinting is used. Bioprinting is layer-by-layer depositing of biological material with living cells using computer-aided transfer processes. Although whole vascularized organs for transplantation have not been produced by bioprinting yet, generation of the scaffold-free tubular trachea [29] and generation of scaffold-free nerve constructs using human gingiva-derived mesenchymal stem cell spheroids were reported [30]. 3-D bioprinting has been used in the production and transplantation of several organs including tracheal splints, vascular grafts, cartilaginous structures, heart tissue, multi-layered skin, and bone. The final goal is industrial bioproduction of individualized functional 3D organs for clinical application.

Nanotechnology has been useful for localized, sustained, and controlled delivery of drugs including immunosuppressive agents and clinically relevant biomarkers. Nano particles can also be used to deliver contrast agents to assist in delineating anatomy and therefore nanotechnology contributes to imaging of clinically relevant biomarkers and functional parameters for diagnosis and treatment [31].

Gene therapy has the potential to eliminate problems associated with immunosuppression by allowing the production of immunomodulatory proteins in the donor grafts resulting in local immunosuppression. Gene therapy may also prevent chronic rejection [32].

5.4 Machine perfusion

Machine perfusion is a novel technique aimed to increased use of suboptimal grafts and consequently to enlarge donor pool. Large animal experiments have revealed the superiority of machine preservation. The possibility of perfusing high-risk livers consistently for 24 hours has been shown. During that period little evidence of deterioration of the functional and histologic characteristics of the livers were noted. It has been claimed that perfusion may overcome the time limitations related with utilization of high risk livers. Another advantage of normothermic machine perfusion is measuring the functional parameters which give an idea about the viability of the organ [33] and this feature of machine perfusion is also valid for heart. The clinician may predict the risk of primary graft dysfunction. Repair and conditioning of thoracic organs are at experimental level for the time being. It has been reported that machine perfusion may also act as an immunoregulatory agent for lung [34]. Hypothermic and normothermic machine perfusion and controlled oxygenated rewarming keep kidney grafts functionally and metabolically active during preservation. Ex-vivo kidney perfusion has found clinical practice and on the other hand, preclinical results reveal that prolonged warm perfusion appears superior than a brief end-ischemic reconditioning as far as renal function and injury is concerned [35].

6. Specific organs

6.1 Liver

The liver has vital functions including plasma protein synthesis, hormone production, detoxification, decomposition of red blood cells, and regulation of glycogen storage. Due to these important functions, liver failure poses a threat to life. Historically, liver transplantation is second to kidney transplantation. Liver transplantation is a definitive treatment modality for acute liver failure and end-stage chronic liver disease. The shortage of organ supply has initiated the usage of new therapeutic systems to reduce mortality and bridge patients to transplantation.

Albumin dialysis, plasmapheresis, column perfusion, and hybrid devices are among the instruments that have been used to compensate for liver function.

Artificial liver support systems may replace the failing functions of the organ and therefore time is gained for liver regeneration or transplantation. Artificial liver support systems are expected to detoxify, replenish plasma proteins, and reverse the inflammatory process. Among the artificial liver support systems, molecular adsorbent recirculating system [MARS], therapeutic plasma exchange [TPE], single- pass albumin dialysis [SPAD], and Prometheus can be named. MARS uses albumin dialysis to replace the detoxification function of the liver while TPE improves survival in patients with acute liver failure. MARS and TPE improve systemic hemodynamics and the grade of hepatic encephalopathy [36, 37].

Extracorporeal liver support systems are either cell- based [biological] or non-cell-based. Non- cell-based systems include high volume plasma exchange and albumin dialysis. Bioartificial liver systems improve neurologic function, reduce intracranial pressure and increase cerebral perfusion pressure Biological extracorporeal liver support systems aim to support the failing liver through detoxification [38].

Shen Yi and colleagues have performed a time-series-based meta-analysis of randomized clinical trials and observational studies that examined differences in mortality in acute-on-chronic liver failure patients treated with artificial liver support systems. The results revealed that an artificial liver support system had reduced the risk of short-term [1–3 months] mortality for patients with acute-on-chronic liver failure by nearly 30%. As the results of the meta-analysis suggested, an artificial liver support system might reduce medium-term [6 month-1 year] mortality risk by 30% and long-term [3 years] mortality risk by 50% in acute-on-chronic liver failure patients [39].

The parenchymal cells of the liver are hepatocytes that constitute nearly 70–85% of the liver volume. Treatment of congenital metabolic disorders affecting the liver and acute liver failure using allogenic hepatocyte transplantation has been proposed. The transplanted cells provide the impaired or missing hepatic function once engrafted into the recipient's liver. Mature hepatocytes have been considered the most obvious cell type for liver cell transplantation. Some advantages of these cells have been noted. They are less invasive and less expensive not involving complex surgery, may be repeated in case of need, cryopreserved cells isolated from donor livers are immediately possible when required and native liver stays in place [40].

Demetriou AA et al. have shown favorable results on survival in patients with acute liver failure using an extracorporeal liver assist system. The system was composed of 7 billion porcine hepatocytes within a hollow-fiber bioreactor. This phase II/III, prospective, randomized, multicenter, controlled trial included patients with fulminant-subfulminant hepatic failure or primary nonfunction [41].

6.2 Kidney

Long-term hemodialysis and peritoneal dialysis have been widely used in the treatment of end-stage renal failure patients. These treatment modalities have bridged thousands of patients to transplantation. The kidney is the first solid organ whose function could be replaced by an external device. Portable and wearable dialysis devices for the treatment of patients with end-stage kidney failure are being developed.

The evolution of devices designed to treat renal impaired patients has followed the sequence of portable artificial kidney [PAK], second- generation PAK, a wearable artificial kidney [WAK], and implantable bioartificial kidney [BAK]. All of these devices are to be smaller, lighter and intended for use outside the clinic. BAK can partially replace tubular function and it provides an extension to conventional dialysis systems and artificial kidneys by incorporating elements of living cellular and tissue function. The key features for the development of a bioengineered kidney require three main components. These are, cellular components, material engineering, and emerging technologies. Hollow membranes, extracellular matrix proteins, porous structures, and novel chemistries are included in material engineering. Organoids, 3D printing, decellularized kidney and induced pluripotent stem cells compose the emerging technologies. Specialized kidney cells and stem cells constitute the cellular component. A bioartificial kidney is expected to be able to reproduce the metabolic, endocrine, immunomodulatory, and secretory functions of a normal kidney [42].

Bioengineering and regenerative medicine also play a role in the efforts to construct an artificial kidney as a final target. New branches of engineering like artificial intelligence and machine learning for the real-time analysis of equipment alarm, dialysis parameters and patient-related data contribute to developments in this field. The problems encountered in the transplantation of recellularized whole kidney scaffolds are needed to efficiently repopulate the endothelium of the vascular network of the engineered kidney before implantation and optimal source of cells to repopulate an acellular kidney scaffold [43].

Generation of human- induced pluripotent stem cells derived kidney organoids has been an important step in regenerative medicine and kidney organoids are expected to be used for disease modeling, drug discovery and ultimately be applicable for transplant [44].

6.3 Heart

Left ventricular assist device [LVAD] was developed as mechanical circulatory support [MCS] for heart failure patients. A long-term implantable continuous-flow LVAD named “the Heart II™ left Ventricular Assist system [Abbott Laboratories] has been approved by U.S. Food and Drug Administration for indications of destination therapy and bridging to transplantation. While the technology is advancing to achieve smaller size and eradication of drive lines, the expectation is to apply continuous-flow technology, which is in the experimental phase, to total heart replacement [45].

Implantation of a total artificial heart is indicated in end-stage heart failure patients. Acute hemodynamic restoration and clinical stabilization are achieved and the patient is then bridged to transplantation. It has been reported that a total artificial heart is associated with a post-transplantation survival rate very similar to national survival rates five years after transplantation [46] It has also been reported that total artificial heart patients have high rates of successful bridge-to-transplant and survival on par with biventricular assist device supported patients. The future objectives are decreased device size, continuous flow mechanisms, and use of bioprosthetic materials. Overcoming these hurdles will provide increased device longevity and decreased post-implant complications [47].

Taylor and associates have claimed that engineering a bioartificial heart has become a possibility. They have proposed a novel type of in vivo organ engineering utilizing pre-clinical models where decellularized hearts are heterotopically transplanted. The aim was to harness the capability of the body at least partly to repopulate the scaffold. The authors have added load and electric input and have posited that vascular and parenchymal cell maturation can occur. The authors have implanted porcine decellularized hearts acutely and chronically in living recipients in a heterotopic position and have demonstrated that short-term implantation promotes endothelial cell adhesion to the vessel lumens and that long-term implantation also promotes tissue formation with evidence of cardiomyocytes and endothelial cells present within the graft [48].

Pelletier et al. have reported that Rein-Heart-total artificial heart had shown safe and effective function in vivo and in vitro testing. The Rein-Heart has effectively replaced the native hearts’ functions in animals for up to two days [49].

There are obstacles to overcome before obtaining a bioartificial heart. These obstacles are, achieving adequate durability, longer than five years, minimizing thromboemboli and hemolysis, better efficiency, maintaining pulmonary-systemic circulatory balance and reduced size to accommodate in women and small adolescents and children [50].

6.4 Lung

The structure of the lung is complex and lung decellularization is a complex process. The information is not sufficient. The most suitable cell types, media, and growth factors and how to provide the optimal conditions of ventilation, perfusion and oxygenation along the process of biofabrication are issues to be studied for further progress.

The key problem in producing a bioengineered lung is how to drive stem cell differentiation onto the different cell phenotypes. The role played by physical stimuli is also important in lung bioengineering because the cells within the organ are physiologically subjected to two main stimuli. These stimuli are ventilation and blood perfusion across the organ [51].

Extracorporeal membrane oxygenation and mechanical can be used temporarily as a bridge to transplantation. Experimental transplantation of bioartificial lung developed by perfusion decellularized synthetic scaffolds has been shown to provide gas exchange in vivo over a long period. The present level of achievements reveals that obtaining a transplantable artificial lung is not possible soon [52].

6.5 Pancreas

Artificial pancreas treatment is an alternative treatment that combines insulin pump and continuous glucose monitoring with a control algorithm to deliver insulin in a glucose- responsive manner. It is also named "closed-loop system" or "automated insulin delivery". The artificial pancreas can be either insulin-only or dual hormone [glucagon] type. A systemic review and meta-analysis conducted by Bekiari and associates have shown that artificial pancreas systems are beneficial and safe treatment options for patients with type 1 diabetes. The authors have noted that the current research evidence on artificial pancreas systems is limited by inconsistency in outcome reporting, small sample size, and short follow-up duration of individual trials. So the future efforts should focus on such issues along with exploring artificial pancreas use in relevant groups of people with type 2 diabetes such as those with inpatient hyperglycemia [53]. Other areas of interest for the future would be faster acting insulin in the artificial pancreas, increased accuracy, and reduced lag-time of continuous glucose monitoring. Self-learning adapting algorithms will improve the level of automation and effectiveness. Cost-effectiveness in the general public is another issue to be taken into consideration [54].

7. Conclusion

The basic indication for solid organ transplantation is the treatment of end-stage diseases posing threat to life. Solid- organ transplantation evolved to be gold standard therapy and became a routine procedure with minimal morbidity and mortality figures. Despite the achievements in different fields of transplantation activities, the gap between demand and supply is growing due to an increased percentage of the elderly population, and the increase in the number patients that require organ transplant from which considerable number are lost while awaiting a suitable organ. The unmatched shortage of organs and life-long dependency on immunosuppressive drugs and related complications of immunosuppression had warranted the development of alternative novel technologies for the repair or replacement of missing or malfunctioning organs.

Reproductive, functional, restorative, and psychologic indications have caused the emerging of transplanting different organs, namely face, extremity, and uterus. It is apparent that transplant procedures of these organs will be performed with increasing frequency in the future because successful results are closely associated with the accumulation of useful scientific data and experience.

The unmet demand for organs and the failure of immunosuppressive drugs to prolong long-term graft survival and a variety of complications associated with immunosuppression have caused the need for completely new therapeutic modalities in the treatment of diseased and malfunctioning organs.

For the time being, human grafts and artificial devices are not capable of performing all the functions of vital organs. Artificial devices are beneficial in bridging patients to transplantation, or organ regeneration or as independent implantable units. The ultimate goal is to obtain human grafts to be totally restored in all their structural and functional aspects, and artificial devices that can completely replace native organs. The hurdles on the way can be overcome by close cooperation and integration of a wide variety of disciplines and technologies including tissue engineering, regenerative medicine, electronics, robotics, artificial intelligence, machine learning, 3D bioartificial printing, bioreactor technology, nano- technology, gene therapy, machine perfusion and cell biology. In light of the recent scientific developments, it can easily be assumed that reaching the goals mentioned is a matter of time. Tissue-engineered products and any kind of device expected to substitute totally human organs must certainly be safe, long durable, and non-immune. The cost-effectiveness and the ease of accessibility are issues to be managed in the future.

Author details

Mehmet Nur Altinörs
Department of Neurosurgery, Acıbadem Ankara Hospital, Ankara, Turkey

*Address all correspondence to: mnaltinors@gmail.com

IntechOpen

© 2020 The Author(s). Licensee IntechOpen. This chapter is distributed under the terms of the Creative Commons Attribution License (http://creativecommons.org/licenses/by/3.0), which permits unrestricted use, distribution, and reproduction in any medium, provided the original work is properly cited.

References

[1] Weissenbacher A, Vrakes G, Hasralla D, Ceresa CD: The future of organ perfusion and re-conditioning. Transplant Int. 2019; 32[6]: 586-597.

[2] Argani H: Cell therapy in Solid-Organ transplant. Exp Clin Transplant. 2016; 14 [SUppl 3] 6-13.

[3] Cooper DKC, Ekser B, Tector AJ: A brief History of Clinical Xenotransplantaion. Int J Surg. 2015; 23 [Pt B]: 205-210.

[4] John M, Bailey LL: Neonatal heart transplantation. Ann Cardiothoac Surg. 2018; 7[1]:118-125.

[5] Stolf NAG: Xenotransplantation: on the way to Clinical Application ? Braz J Cardiovasc Surg. 2019; 34[3]:2,

[6] Lu T,Yang B, Wang R, Qin C:Xenotransplantation: Current Status in Preclinical Research. Front Immunol, 2020; 23;10:3060.

[7] Ekser B, Li P, Cooper DKC: Xenotransplantaton: Past, Present and Future. Curr Opin Organ Transplant. 2017; 22[6]: 513-521.

[8] Pitkin Z: New Phase of Growth for Xenogeneic-Based Bioartificial organs. Int J Mol Sci. 2016; 17[9]:1593.

[9] Gilbert R. Hand transplanted from cadaver is reamputated.Med Trib Med News. 1964;5:23-25.

[10] Dubernard JM, Owen E, Herzberg G, Lanzetta M, Martin X, Kapilla H, Dawahra M, Hakim NS: Human hand allograft:report on first 6 months. Lancet. 1999; 353 [9161]:1315-1320.

[11] Dubernard JM, Petruzzo P, Lanzetta M, Parmentier H, Martin X, Dawahra M, Hakim NS, Owen E. Functional results of the human double-hand transplantation. Ann Surg. 2003; 238[1]: 128-136.

[12] Salminger S, Sturma A, Roche AD, Hruby LA, Paternostro-Sluga T, Kumnig M et al.: Functional and psychosocial outcomes of hand transplantation compared with prosthetic fitting in below-elbow amputees: a multicenter cohort study. PLos One.2016; 11[9]:e0162507.

[13] Eun SC: Facial Transplantation Surgery Introduction. J Korean Med Sci. 2015 30[6]: 669-672.

[14] Lee ZH, Lopez CD, Plana NM, Caplan AL, Rodriguez ED: Are we prepared for the inevitable ? A survey on Defining and Managing Failure in Face Transplantation: Plast Reconstr Surg Glob Open. 2019; 7[5]:e2055.

[15] Petruzzo P, Testelin S, Kantakis J,Badet L, Lengelé B, Girbon JP, Permentier H, Malcus C, Morelon E, Devauchelle B, Bubernard JM: First human face transplantation: 5 years outcomes. Transplantation. 2012;93:236-240.

[16] Petruzzo P, Kantakis J, Testelin S, Pialat JB, Buron F, Badet L et al.: Clinicopathologic findings of chronic rejection in a face grefted patient. Transplantation. 2015; 99[12]:2644-2650.

[17] Özkan Ö, Özkan Ö, Doğan U, Yılmaz VT, Uysal H, Ündar L et al.: Considerations of difficulties and exit strategies in a case of face allotransplantation resulting in failure. Microsurgery. 2017; 37[6]:661-668.

[18] Lubek JE: Facial transplantation: what does the future hold? Oral Surg Oral Med Oral Pathol Oral Radiol. 2019; 128[4]:345-346.

[19] Eraslan S, Hamernik RJ, Hardy JD: Replantation of uterus and ovaries in

dogs with successful pregnancy. Arch Surg. 1966; 92[1]:9-12.

[20] Nair A, Stega J, Smith JR,Del Priore G. Uterus transplant:evidence and ethics. Ann N Y Acad Sci. 2008; 1127:83-91.

[21] Akar EM, Ozkan O, Aydinuraz B, Dirican K, Cincik M, Mendilcioğlu I: Clinical pregnancy after uterus transplantation. Fertil Steril. 2013; 100[5]:1358-1363.

[22] Brännström M, Johannesson L, Bokström H,Kvarnström N, Mölne J, Dahm-Kahler P, Enskog A, Milenkovic M, Ekberg J, Diaz-Garcia C,Gäbel M, Hanafy A,Hagberg H, Olaussan M, Nilsson L: Livebirth after uterus transplantation. Lancet 2015;385[9968]:607-616.

[23] Lefkowitz A, Edwards M, Balayla J: The Montral Criteria for the Ethical Feasibility of Uterus Transplanatation. Transplant Int. 2012; 25[4]:439-447.

[24] Hillebrandt KH, Everwien H, Haep N, Keshi E, Pratschke J, Sauer IM: Strategies based on organ cellularization and recellularization. Transplant Int. 2019; 32[6]: 571-585.

[25] Orlando G, Soker S, Stratte RJ, Atala A: Will Regenerative Medicine Replace Transplantation ? Cold Spring Harb Perspect Med. 2013; 1;3[8]:a015693.

[26] Porzionato A, Stocco E, Barbon S, Grandi F, Macchi V, deCaro R: Tissue-Engineered Grafts from Human Decellularized Extracellular Matrices: A Systematic Review and future Perspectives. Int J Mol Sci. 2018; 19[12]:4117.

[27] Messner F, Guo Y, Etra JW, Brandacher G: Emerging technologies in organ preservation, tissue engineering and regenerative medicine: a blessing or curse for transplantation ? Transplant Int. 2019; 32[7]: 673-685.

[28] Wang X: Bioartificial organ manufacturing Technologies. Cell Transplant. 2019; 28[1]: 5-17.

[29] Taniguchi D, Matsumoto K, Tsuchiya T, Machino R, Yosuke T, Elgalad A et al.: Scaffold-free trachea regeneration by tissue engineering with bio-3D printing. Interact Cardiovasc Thorac Surg. 2018; 26[5]:745-752.

[30] Zhang Q, Nguyen PD, Shi S, Burrell JC, Cullen DK, Le AD: 3D bio-printed scaffold-free nerve constructs with human gingiva-derived mesenchymal stem cells promote rat facial nerve regeneration. Sci Rep. 2018; 8[1]: 6634.

[31] Tasciotti E, Cabrera FJ, Evangelopoulos M, Martinez JO, Thekkedath UR, Kloc M et al.: The emerging role of nanotechnology in cell and organ transplantation. Transplantation. 2016; 100[8]: 1629-1638.

[32] Bagley J, Jacomini J: Gene therapy progress and prospects: gene therapy in organ transplantation. GeneTher. 2003; 10[8]:605-611.

[33] Vogel T, Brockmann JG, Quaglia A, Morovat A, Jassem W, Heaton ND, Coussios CC, Friend PJ: The 24-hour normothermic machine perfusion of discarded human liver grafts. Liver Transplant. 2017; 23(2):207-220

[34] Van Raemdonck D, Rega F, Rex S, Neyrinck A: Machine perfusion of thoracic organs. J Thorac Dis. 2018; 10(Suppl 8): S910-S923

[35] Hamar M, Selzner M: Ex-vivo machine perfusion for kidney preservation. Curr Opin Organ Transplant. 2018; 23(3): 369-374

[36] Saliba F, Samuel D: Artificial Liver Support: A Real Step Forward. Minerva Med. 2015 106[1]:35-43,

[37] Larsen FS: Artificial LÎver Support in Acute and Acute-On-Chronic Liver

Failure. Curr Opin Crit Care. 2019; 25[2]:187-191.

[38] Karvellas CJ, Subramanian RM: Current Evidence for Extracorporeal Liver Support Systems in Acute Liver Failure and Acute-on-Chronic Liver Failure. Crit Care Clin. 2016; 32[3]: 439-451.

[39] Shen Y, Wang XL, Wang B, Shae JG, Liu YM, Qin Y et al.: Survival benefits With Artificial Liver Support System for Acute-on-Chronic Liver Failure: A Time Series-Based Meta Analysis. Medicine [Baltimore]. 2016; 95[3]:e2506.

[40] Iansante V, Mitry RR, Filippi C, Fitzpatrick E, Dhavan A: Human hepatocyte transplantation for liver disease: current status and future perspectives. Ped Res. 2018; 83 [1-2]: 232-240.

[41] Demetriou AA, Brown RS Jr, Busuttil RW, Fair J, McGuire BM, Rosenthal P et al.: Prospective, Randomized, Multicenter, Controlled Trial of Bioartificial Liver in Treating Acute Failure. Ann Surg. 2004; 239[5]: 660-670.

[42] van Gelder MK, Mihalia SM, Jansen J, Wester M, Verhaar MC, Joles JA et al.: From portable dialysis to a bioengineered kidney. Exp Rev Med Dev. 2018; 15[5]: 323-336.

[43] Hueso M, Navarro E, Sandoval D, Cruzado JM: Progress in the development and challanges for the use of Artificial Kidneys and Wearable Dialysis Devices. Kidney [Basel]. 2019; 5[1]: 3-10.

[44] Naganuma H, Nishinakamura R: From organoids to transplantable artificial kidneys. Transplant Int. 2019; 32[6]: 563-570.

[45] Alnajar A, Frazier OH: The State of Artificial Heart Therapy. Tex Heart Inst J. 2019; 46[1]: 77-79.

[46] Copeland JG, Smith RG, Arabia RG, Nolan PE, Sethi GK et al.: Cardiac Replacement with a Total Artificial Heart as a Bridge to Transplantation. N Eng J Med. 2004; 26; 351[9]: 859-867.

[47] Beaupre RA, Frazier OH, Morgan JA: Total artificial heart implantation as a bridge to transplantation: a viable model for the future? Expert Rev Med Devices. 2018; 15[10]:710-706.

[48] Taylor DA, Frazier OH, Elgalad A, Hochman-Mendez C, Sampaio LC: Building a Total Bioartificial Heart. Harnessing Nature to overcome the Current Hurdles. Artif Organs. 2018; 42[10]:970-982.

[49] Pelletier B, Spiliopoulos S, Finocchiaro T, Graef F, Kuipers K et al.: System overview of the fully implantable destination therapy-Rein Heart-total artificial heart. Eur J Cardiothoracic Surg. 2015; 47[1]: 80-86.

[50] Hulman M, Artemiou P, Hudec V, Olejarova I, Goncalvesova E: SynCardia, total artificial heart as a bridge to transplant. Bratislava Med J. 2019; 120[5]:325-330.

[51] Nonaka PN, Uriarte JJ, Campillo N, Oliveira VR, Navajas D, Farre R: Lung bioengineering: physical stimuli and stem/progenitor cell biology towards biofabricating a functional organ. Respir Res, 2016; 28; 17[1]: 161.,

[52] Petrella F, Spaggiari L: Artificial lung. J Thorac Di. 2018;s 10 [Suppl 20]:S2329-S2332.

[53] Bekiari E, Kitsios K, Thabit H, Tauschmann M, Athanasiadou E, Karagiannis T et al.: Artificial pancreas treatment for outpatients with type 1 diabetes ,systemic review and meta-analysis.BMJ. 2018; 18;361:k1310.

[54] Ramli R, Reddy M, Oliver N: Artificial Pancreas: Current Progress and Future Outlook in the Treatment of Type 1 Diabetes. Drugs. 2019; 79[10] 1089-1101.